Claire. P. BURRIDGE

Physiother

PHYSIOTHERAPY IN PSYCHIATRY

by

Mary Hare

Senior Physiotherapist, Hinchingbrooke Hospital, Huntingdon

Foreword by Lois Dyer OBE. MCSP

HEINEMANN PHYSIOTHERAPY

First published in 1986
by William Heinemann Medical Books
23 Bedford Square, London WC1B 3HH

© Mary Hare, 1986

ISBN 0 433 13280 9

Filmset by Wilmaset, Birkenhead, Wirral
Printed in Great Britain by
Biddles Limited, Guildford

Contents

Preface		vii
Acknowledgements		ix
Foreword by Lois Dyer OBE, MCSP		xi
Chapter 1.	An Introduction to Mental Health Care	1
2.	The Classification of Mental Illness – Some Common Terms Explained	6
3.	Physiotherapy in Acute Mental Illness	12
4.	Chronic Mental Illness	41
5.	Mental Illness in the Elderly	66
6.	Psychiatric Drugs and Their Side-effects	94
7.	Techniques for the Relief of Stress	108
8.	Working in Specialist Units	129
9.	The Physiotherapy Department and its Management in a Mental Health Care Setting	157
	Appendix I	174
	Appendix II	183
	Index	185

Preface

In recent years there has been a growing tendency for the physiotherapist to be regarded as a necessary member of the mental health care team rather than a health care professional called in to treat isolated cases of physical disability occurring in the mentally ill. A number of factors have contributed to this, including the increasing numbers of mentally ill elderly people, an emphasis on community care for the mentally ill, the recognition of the value of relaxation, exercise and self help techniques as an alternative to reliance on habit forming drugs and a more general awareness of the importance of the relationship between mind and body.

Those physiotherapists already working in the field of psychiatry in the United Kingdom have responded to the need for a more informed approach to the care of the mentally ill by forming a Special Interest Group of the Chartered Society of Physiotherapy. The result of this has been a pooling of information and expertise and the holding of regular courses in various aspects of physiotherapy involvement in psychiatric care. A small number of relevant articles have recently been published but, as physiotherapists working in the community and in district general hospitals come into increasing contact with the mentally ill, there has been no book of reference available.

A family move necessitated resignation from my job at Fulbourn Hospital, Cambridge and I decided that rather than return to work immediately I would write this book. I have attempted to write the type of book I would have wanted to read when my colleague and I, both with no previous experience in caring for the mentally ill, were faced with the problem of establishing an active physiotherapy service in a large psychiatric hospital. The book is designed to give a comprehensive overview of the range of physiotherapy involvement in mental health care, together with a very basic grounding in clinical psychiatry.

I have not recommended specific treatments for specific conditions, but have rather suggested a variety of ways in which problems may be approached, illustrating these with case histories which highlight not only the successes but some of the pitfalls when treating the mentally ill. Flexibility in the approach to treatment and the methods used is of the essence in the field of psychiatry, and the physiotherapist who is a good generalist and who is willing to teach and be taught by other members of the mental health care team is most likely to succeed. Two other points are worth mentioning, first that a chapter on community physiotherapy in psychiatry has not been possible because this field is so much in its infancy that there is as yet an inadequate overview of the subject and second that throughout the book the physiotherapist is referred to as 'she' and the patient as 'he'. This is solely to aid the flow of the text for the reader and is not intended to be sexist.

I hope that this book will be of value to many physiotherapists, not only those working with the mentally ill, but those who encounter incidental mental illness in their patients. I trust it will also be of use to other members of mental health care teams concerned with the physical well being of the mentally ill. Above all I hope that, by contributing towards the better care of the whole patient, this book will benefit those who suffer from any form of mental illness.

Mary Hare, 1986

Acknowledgements

I could not have written this book without the help of many others. Some have generously donated hours of time to helpful comment and criticism, others may not have realised the value of their ideas expressed in the course of conversation or correspondence.

My special thanks goes to Dr Richard Latcham, Consultant Psychiatrist to the Huntingdon District Health Authority for his painstaking and patient advice on the presentation of the clinical psychiatry in the book. My colleagues Mrs Margaret Webb (MCSP) and Mrs Susan Fox (MCSP) and the members of the Division of Psychiatry of Fulbourn Hospital, Cambridge are gratefully thanked for their support and for permission to publish the case histories.

Many others willingly gave me help and amongst these I would very much like to thank Mrs E. Ricketts (MCSP) of Whitchurch Hospital, Cardiff, Mrs H. Hayward (MCSP) and Dr A. Minto of Rampton Hospital, Mrs J. Freeman (MCSP) and Mrs J. Abbott (MCSP) of the Towers Hospital, Leicester and the committee and members of the Association of Chartered Physiotherapists in Psychiatry.

My family have been very supportive during the writing of this book. My children Katy, Rachael, Pippa and Thomas have innocently boosted my morale by their obvious delight in the idea of a mother who has written a book, but I owe most thanks to my husband John who first encouraged me to write and then selflessly ensured that I should have all the time, advice and emotional support I needed to carry the project through.

Mary Hare, 1986

Foreword

Until recently, most physiotherapists appear to have ignored or, at best, underrated the value of their skills in helping those suffering from mental disorders or illness. The pioneering work of Mrs Hare and fellow physiotherapists has done much to remedy this state of affairs. They have demonstrated to colleagues in their own and allied professions that physiotherapists have a useful contribution to make in this neglected field.

Consequently, increased interest is being shown by qualified and student physiotherapists, but little has been written to offer appropriate guidance. Recognising the need, Mrs Hare has produced a book which covers a complex and sometimes controversial subject. The references and bibliography provide a valuable source for further reading and study.

Quite rightly, it is accepted that measures used to treat physical problems of psychiatric patients vary little from those used when treating any patients with physiotherapy. The author stresses the importance of a basic understanding of the most common mental disorders and illnesses, and the way in which this might influence the approach and clinical judgement of the physiotherapist. The use of case histories should appeal to readers who will feel familiar with many of the problems presented.

The challenge of ever increasing demands for a physiotherapy service calls for a reassessment of the traditional allocation of resources to meet the needs of patients. This is a reality in the fields of both physical and mental illness. Sensibly, Mrs Hare emphasises the teaching and supportive role of physiotherapists for patients and those who care for them.

The part which physiotherapists might usefully play in

prevention of problems at primary, secondary and tertiary levels has yet to be explored and here there is surely a place for physiotherapy in psychiatry.

This area of work, new to so many physiotherapists, offers a unique opportunity for evaluation and research. Accurate observation and recording can provide data to examine the value of their contribution.

This book constitutes a landmark in the development of physiotherapy and is a tribute to those who have had the foresight and courage to promote ways in which physiotherapists might meet the historically unrecognised needs of an important group of the population.

Lois Dyer OBE, MCSP

1

An Introduction to Mental Health Care

The Historical Background to Mental Health Care in the United Kingdom

The care of the mentally ill has evolved separately from the care of the physically ill and it is necessary to know a little of the historical background of mental health care in order to understand current attitudes to the mentally ill.

Until the beginning of the nineteenth century in the United Kingdom the terms of the Poor Law, Vagrancy and Mad House Acts resulted in lunatics being locked up in mad houses, workhouses and prisons, in appalling conditions with no hope of release or treatment. Such people were even displayed to the general public as a ghoulish peep show. At the beginning of the nineteenth century, asylums were built out in the country with the then enlightened aim of providing more humane care for the mentally ill. Many of these buildings are still in use as mental hospitals throughout the United Kingdom. The detention of the mad, and sometimes the not so mad, in these asylums was governed by a series of Acts, the most important of which was the Lunacy Act of 1890 whereby no patient could be admitted to a mental hospital except by a magistrate's order. Increasing numbers of patients were admitted to asylums, and while some institutions struggled to remain humane others deteriorated into overcrowded prisons where patients spent their whole lives in squalid conditions out of sight of the general public. This was the case until 1930 when the Mental Treatment Act at last paved the way to allowing patients to be admitted voluntarily to a mental institution for treatment.

When the 1959 Mental Health Act became law in

England and Wales, certification by a magistrate was abolished and compulsory admissions to a mental hospital became a medical problem rather than a matter for a court of law. The 1959 Mental Health Act was responsible for removing much of the stigma surrounding mental illness and as a result the number of compulsory admissions to mental institutions has fallen to about 10% of total admissions.

In Scotland it is still the case that the Procurator Fiscal has to ratify compulsory orders made by social workers and doctors. There are many who consider that this is a better system than the English one, in that it provides lay control over the compulsory admission of patients.

The Mental Health Act of 1983

Modern legislation governing the care of the mentally ill in England and Wales is founded on the Mental Health Act of 1959, and its subsequent amendments in 1982 and 1983. Four further amendment acts are planned.

The aims of the Mental Health Act of 1983 are, amongst other things, to enable psychiatric patients to have the ability to appeal against compulsory detention and treatment in a more practical way. The new act is complicated and legislatively covers the following four categories:

Mental impairment
Severe mental impairment
Mental illness
Psychopathic disorder.

Alcoholism, drug dependency and sexual deviation are excluded from this act. It should be noted that the treatment of the mentally impaired is beyond the scope of this book.

Strict regulations govern the compulsory admission of a patient to a psychiatric unit, and the detention of a patient under a section of the Mental Health Act of 1983 must be reviewed at specific times. The patient also has rights of appeal to a mental health tribunal.

Mentally ill patients may be detained under one of a number of section orders. Those which the physiotherapist is most likely to see used are:

Section 2, admission for assessment
Section 3, admission for treatment
Section 4, emergency admission
Section 37, a hospital order by a court of law to admit a mentally ill offender found guilty of a crime to a psychiatric hospital
Section 41, a hospital order with a restriction order 'to protect the public from serious harm'. The Home Secretary's consent is needed for the discharge or transfer of these patients.

It should be emphasised that 90% of patients are voluntary and are free to enter and leave hospital for treatment as are patients with physical disorders.

A new Mental Health Act Commission has been established with powers to inspect mental health care units in the United Kingdom. New clauses have been introduced governing consent to treatment and compulsory treatment. This Mental Health Act Commission does not only include doctors but also those who are interested in the welfare, treatment and rights of the mentally ill such as voluntary associations like MIND (National Association for Mental Health).

Readers from countries other than the United Kingdom will of course bear in mind that legislation and the background to psychiatric care in their country will differ from that described.

Current Trends and Policies in Mental Health Care

Mental health care policies are continually under review. At present the emphasis is on treatment within the community rather than removal to isolated specialist hospitals. This attitude runs parallel to plans for the mentally impaired and the physically disabled. Acute wards for the mentally ill are being attached to district general hospitals. Day centres play an increasingly important role in the care of the mentally ill, thus avoiding the need for admission to hospital.

The application of these plans is however not complete, and it is doubtful whether adequate resources are available to provide a comprehensive community service in all these areas for some years. Community physiotherapy is increasing in importance and in demand. The return of large numbers of chronically mentally ill elderly people to the community is a considerable challenge to all members of the community service.

Mentally ill patients with acute physical problems will also in future, find themselves being treated in physiotherapy departments in general hospitals rather than by specialist physiotherapists in psychiatric hospitals. The need for the physiotherapist to know more about mental illness in the future is apparent.

Care of the increasing numbers of mentally ill elderly people is a great problem for both the present and the future, and is discussed in Chapter 5.

Physiotherapy Involvement in Mental Health Care

Historically there has been little involvement in the care of the mentally ill by physiotherapists. The early forms of custodial care were introduced long before physiotherapy existed as a profession. During the period after the Mental Health Act of 1959, the emphasis in psychiatric hospitals was on freedom for the patient, improving the quality of life and of course, treating the mind. Physical disabilities received little professional attention.

Once again ideas are changing and, coupled with an emphasis on community care, an interest is growing in the relationship between mind and body and the effect each has on the other. It is now realised that some of the skills that the physiotherapist has to offer in the areas of exercise therapy and relaxation instruction are as effective as drug therapy without the side-effects.

Until recently the teaching of any form of psychiatry in schools of physiotherapy had been non-existent. Now it is minimal. The addition of basic psychology to the syllabus is comparatively recent. As a result, the majority of qualified physiotherapists are as ignorant of the nature of mental illness as the general public. Nevertheless, the physiotherapist may be called on to treat a suicidal patient with a self-inflicted injury, a patient with an anxiety neurosis and backache, or an old lady becoming immobile with senile dementia.

There is a need for all physiotherapists to have a working knowledge of the major mental illnesses and their effects. This need is becoming increasingly acute as the large Victorian asylums are disbanded. In addition, some physiotherapists who are particularly interested in the care of the mentally ill will find a place for themselves in all areas of mental health care. Consequently, there is much scope for research into physiotherapy in mental health.

Further Reading

Bluglass R. S. (1984). *A Guide to the Mental Health Act 1983*. Edinburgh: Churchill Livingstone.

Goffman E. (1972). *Asylums*. New York: Anchor Books, Doubleday and Colne.

Jones W. L. (1983). *Ministering to Minds Diseased*. London: William Heinemann Medical Books.

Partridge C. J. (1984). *Community Physiotherapy and Direct Access to Physiotherapy Services by General Practitioners within the NHS*. London: King's College.

Scull A. T. (1982). The social organisation of insanity in Nineteenth Century England. In *Museums of Madness*. Harmondsworth: Penguin Books.

2

The Classification of Mental Illness – Some Common Terms Explained

The older textbooks of psychiatry classify mental illnesses into neat categories of disease, thus attempting to provide easily recognisable medical models. In practice the boundaries in mental illness are frequently less easy to define. Nowadays much broader classifications are used and all the time the interplay between different types of mental illness in the same patient is carefully considered.

Psychoses and Neuroses

The term **psychosis** infers that a patient's illness is causing a distortion of perception. Psychotic disorders of mood and of thinking can also occur.

The term **neuroses** refers to disorders which present as understandable exaggerations of normal behaviour or emotion in the context of external circumstances.

General Classification of Mental Illness

The Psychoses

The psychoses are subdivided as follows:

Functional Psychoses

Many factors have been imputed in the genesis of these psychoses including both genetic and environmental factors.

Schizophrenia
Manic depressive psychosis (affective psychosis)

Organic Psychoses

Organic psychoses have a definable physical origin. They affect the normal function of the brain either in the short term or permanently.

Acute organic psychoses involve acute confusion of the brain and can also be termed delirium. Typical causes are: severe infection; brain trauma; cerebral anoxia; intoxication by, or withdrawal from, alcohol or drugs.

Chronic organic psychoses These conditions produce permanent brain damage, typical examples include: degeneration, for example, Alzheimer's disease; Huntington's chorea; drugs and alcohol, for example, alcoholic dementia; neoplasm; trauma; epilepsy. (Only the severest forms of epilepsy are included here, most epileptics are not under the care of psychiatrists and lead normal lives with the help of drug therapy.)

The Neuroses

The neuroses are often related to stress and physical and emotional circumstances, the different disorders may occur separately or combined with other forms of mental disorder. Those disorders which primarily affect the mood are termed affective disorders.

Neurotic depression
Anxiety states
Phobias
Hysteria
Obsessive compulsive states

Personality disorders

Eating disorders (Such as anorexia nervosa and bulimia).
Sexual disorders
Alcohol abuse and drug addiction

Mental impairment (Mental handicap)

Psychosomatic Disorders

Psychosomatic disorders are not discussed in detail in this book. They are physical illnesses which are thought to be partly caused by psychological factors. The term 'psychosomatic' is often misused to infer that a patient's signs and symptoms have been conjured up in his own mind and are not due to physical change.

Physiotherapists working in all areas of their profession are likely to encounter patients with these illnesses. Illnesses in which psychological factors may, in part, have a causative role include:

Asthma, hay fever
Gastrointestinal disorders, for example, ulcers, colitis
Skin conditions, for example, eczema
Rheumatoid arthritis
Cardiovascular disorders, for example, coronary heart disease, hypertension
Menstrual disturbance, for example, premenstrual tension
Endocrine disorders, for example, hyperthyroidism, diabetes mellitus.

Emotional disturbance and major life events have a significant effect on the onset, severity, duration and outcome of these physical illnesses. Medical practitioners are increasingly interested in the factors that influence these illnesses and the increased interest by general practitioners in holistic medicine reflects the importance of psychological factors in the aetiology of some physical illnesses.

Some Common Terms Explained

Psychiatrist. A psychiatrist is a medical practitioner who has postgraduate qualifications enabling him to diagnose and treat mental illness in a specialist capacity. The name is derived from two Greek words, *psyche* meaning mind, spirit or soul and *iatros* meaning physician.

Psychology. Psychology is the study of behaviour and mental activity. The clinical psychologist has a degree in psychology and a higher degree in clinical psychology and works with the psychiatric team. The clinical psychologist is involved in examining the mental background to patients' illnesses using various psychological tests. Nowadays the clinical psychologist is an important member of a multidisciplinary team and is involved in both the treatment of patients and research into all aspects of psychiatry.

Behaviour Therapy. These techniques are usually practised by psychologists, trained nurse therapists and psychiatrists. The methods seek to re-educate patients who are considered to have abnormal learned behaviour patterns. Such behaviour patterns include phobias and obsessional disorders.

Psychotherapy. Psychotherapy is a broad term which includes many types of therapist/patient interaction. Psychotherapy can take several forms: First, it may be supportive during a particular crisis such as bereavement; second, it may be aimed at helping a patient to come to an understanding concerning his current behaviour and thinking in relation to past events of his life. Various hypothetical models exist as a setting in which to carry out such psychotherapy, and many of these models have their origins in Freud's writing. Freud's style of working has been termed psychoanalysis and a therapist involved in such work often uses her relationship with the patient to help in the therapeutic process. For this reason the analyst must understand what she contributes to that relationship, and must therefore have personally experienced psychoanalysis in an extensive period of training.

Psychotherapy may also take the form of group therapy which usually involves groups of about six to ten patients and one or two therapists working together on a regular basis. The way in which individuals in the group interact with each other is used as a reflection of the way in which those individuals may make relationships in their day-to-day living.

Other forms of psychotherapy which are increasingly used in modern psychiatry include family therapy and marital therapy.

Physical Treatments and Physical Methods

In many text books of psychiatry there is a chapter headed 'physical treatments' or 'physical methods'. The uninitiated physiotherapist may hopefully turn to this chapter only to find it has nothing to do with physiotherapy. Physical therapy is probably a more suitable term to use here. The treatments referred to are:

Electroconvulsive Therapy (ECT, Electroplexy, Shock Therapy)

Electroconvulsive therapy or ECT is a treatment in which patients are given therapeutic convulsions (fits) by means of passing an electric current through the brain. The treatment is given under general anaesthesia combined with the administration of a muscle relaxant. The muscle relaxant prevents the risk of injury during a convulsion.

ECT is used as a treatment for certain forms of depression but is less widely used by psychiatrists in the United Kingdom than it used to be. Some sectors of the general public and some doctors have reservations about the use of ECT and in certain states in the United States of America the use of ECT is banned. Although ECT was formerly overprescribed, most psychiatrists would now agree that it is of considerable value in selected cases of psychotic depression. In the United Kingdom where ECT is in regular use, a course of ECT will usually involve twice weekly treatments for three to six weeks. The patient must be fit enough to undergo this number of light general anaesthetics. The patient may experience some amnesia for a short time after each treatment, in the same way as a person who has had an epileptic fit does.

Psychosurgery

The ethical considerations together with poor outcome and high mortality of this form of treatment have made it extremely rare in psychiatric illness. Nevertheless there are still considerable numbers of patients alive who have had such operations and they often present many rehabilitative difficulties in which the physiotherapist may be involved.

Liaison Psychiatry

The increasing awareness of the psychological factors associated with all forms of illness has produced an increase in the provision of psychiatric advice in the care of patients looked after by general practitioners and hospital practitioners. This increased involvement of the psychiatrist in other areas of medicine has been named liaison psychiatry and it requires a close rapport between psychiatrist, hospital specialist and general practitioner in order that both the physical and the psychological aspects of an illness can be assessed jointly.

Further Reading

Kendell R. E., Zealley A. K., eds (1983). *The Companion to Psychiatric Studies*. Edinburgh: Churchill Livingstone.

Priest R., Woolfson G. (1986). *Handbook of Psychiatry (8th ed.)*. London: William Heinemann Medical Books.

Trethowan, Sir William, Sims A. C. P. (1983). *Psychiatry*. Eastbourne, Sussex: Ballière Tindall.

3

Physiotherapy in Acute Mental Illness

The Acute Unit

Units for the treatment of acute mental illness may be found in community day centres, general hospitals and as part of the old style separate psychiatric hospitals. Most units emphasise patient assessment and treatment, with a speedy return to the community and treatment continued in the community rather than in hospital.

The atmosphere of the acute unit is usually informal and friendly; staff and patients may be on first name terms. There is increasing emphasis on the multidisciplinary team as opposed to the old hierarchical system; however, various members of the team, including physiotherapists, who are less often in the unit than others may find it less easy to involve themselves to their full potential.

Doctors and nurses who have had a general medical training will have considerable understanding of physical problems, however a large proportion of psychiatric nurses have not followed a general nurse training and need more advice when physical problems occur in their patients. In addition psychologists, music and art therapists and occupational therapists who have always specialised in mental health care will be less experienced in the care of physical disorders. As a result the physiotherapist, who is able to give simple practical advice on physical problems, will be valued for that role in a ward team. Reciprocally, she must not hesitate to seek advice on a patient's mental state and treatment, in which she may have had no formal training.

The Ward Routine

The ward routine will be supervised by a charge nurse. Patients will be expected, where possible, to organise their own daily toilet, make their own beds, and dress appropriately. A general timetable, with daily activities, is usually prominently displayed. Some activities, such as a regular morning review, require that all patients and ward staff attend, whereas other activities may offer a choice. Within this framework of therapeutic activities, individual patients will be given their own timetables to suit their individual requirements.

General Physiotherapy

Movement sessions

Patients on acute psychiatric wards can spend a great deal of time sitting about. Patients sit during group therapy sessions, on top of which drugs may make them lethargic. A general movement session held regularly as part of the ward routine can help in several ways:

Movement prevents stiffness, keeps the chest clear and maintains basic body functions.
The patient may use movement to express feelings he is unable to put into words.
The contrast of activity helps to stimulate the mood.
Group games promote intercommunication.
The physiotherapist can informally assess the mobility of patients and note any new problems.

There can be no set style for a movement session which will vary according to the needs of the patients and the facilities available. Keep fit, games, free expression and 'music and movement' can all be considered. Other staff should be encouraged to take part and the session could be used by a trained group therapist, who joins in, to invite a discussion afterwards.

As in all psychiatric care, flexibility on the part of the group leader is essential and the wide age range encountered amongst the patients will tax ingenuity. The physiotherapist needs to be alert to the possibility of initiating violence and be skilled in channelling that energy into more positive activity. All mental health care units have a policy on dealing with violence. The physiotherapist must acquaint herself with this and strictly adhere to its guidelines. In addition, the side-effects of drug therapy may impair a patient's physical ability (Chapter 6).

The success or otherwise of the movement group should be discussed at ward meetings.

Small Groups and Individual Work

The subdivision of a ward into smaller groups or individuals could be necessary if, for example, there was an influx of younger patients who needed the stimulation of a greater physical challenge. This group could be offered the opportunity to join in recreational activities such as jogging, circuit training or volley ball with the emphasis on recreation, enjoyment and general fitness rather than physical treatment.

Self Esteem

The physiotherapist can play an important part in increasing a patient's self esteem, particularly in relation to a patient's perception of his own body. Poor posture and general physical debility can contribute to a person's continued belief that they are unwell even after receiving appropriate psychiatric or medical treatment for the original illness. A general improvement in the posture and fitness of the patient does help to increase self esteem. It should also be noted that some patients fear loss of face among their contemporaries if their regular physical recreation prior to illness was particularly competitive. In addition, a person whose posture and general demeanour makes him appear unwell may stimulate acquaintances to comment on the fact; however kindly this is meant, it may reinforce the feeling of being physically unwell.

Case History (3.1)

Mr. *A*, aged 36, was admitted to an acute psychiatric unit from the urology ward of a general hospital where he had been undergoing kidney and bladder function tests. He was severely depressed and threatening suicide. During the previous ten years Mr. *A* had had three operations for the removal of kidney stones from his right kidney. Nine months previously a right nephrectomy had been performed. Mr. *A*'s physical problems coincided with increasing stress and pressure at work and a major setback in his unsuccessful personal life.

Mr. *A*'s depression was complicated by an anxiety state and a hospital phobia as a result of his longstanding urological problems. He was terrified of losing his other kidney, could not bear to be touched or examined and dreaded returning to the urology department for further tests. This anxiety and fear was expressed by complaints of pain, digestive and bladder problems and hyperventilation (*see* Chapter 7). The urologists were particularly hampered by the way in which the anxiety state affected Mr. *A*'s bladder function.

The physiotherapist was asked to join the team working with Mr. *A* and to assess the extent of his physical debility. Mr. *A* reluctantly agreed to this. Initially he was willing only to talk, and over a period of two weeks gradually expressed his total despair as a result of his physical condition. Formerly a keen and successful sportsman, he felt he could never enjoy any form of physical activity again; even the physical demands of daily living were too much.

With many misgivings Mr. *A* began a daily regimen of simple keep fit exercises with the emphasis on improving his round-shouldered posture and moving freely in the space around him. Mr. *A* was encouraged to keep a daily chart of his activity in order to monitor his progress. This treatment scheme was combined with the mental health care team's schedule of individual psychotherapy and group therapy. Gradually it became possible to develop the keep fit routine into a much more vigorous training circuit including weight lifting routines, jogging and use of equipment such as the static bicycle and the rowing machine. During this period Mr. *A* had several emotional setbacks which adversely affected his training programme but the overall physical progress shown in the daily records helped to overcome this.

Mr. A's anxiety state and phobia needed consideration in conjunction with the physical rehabilitation programme. A nurse and the physiotherapist worked together in this field. The physiotherapist taught Mr. A Papworth Hospital breathing exercises and the Laura Mitchell method of tension control (*see* Chapter 7). Mr. A was taught how to utilise these techniques when being touched or interviewed in preparation for further urological investigations. The nurse took Mr. A on practise visits to the general hospital out-patient's department where he also practised the relaxation techniques.

The nurse concerned was a young, very fit man and he also came to some of Mr. A's training sessions and competed in a friendly way with him. Mr. A was very encouraged by his newfound ability to hold his own against someone 10 years his junior.

The physiotherapist began to direct Mr. A's physical activities towards a more recreational approach. He started to play golf again during weekend leave at home and booked some refresher driving lessons in a dual control car. Subsequently Mr. A was able to make a successful visit to the outpatient urology department where he was pronounced fitter than he had been for many years. The whole scheme of treatment had lasted nine months.

Relaxation

The provision of relaxation sessions in a unit can be the province of several professions. Physiotherapists, nurses, doctors, psychologists and occupational therapists all teach relaxation. The professions which teach relaxation vary from one unit to another and tend to be a matter of local tradition. An offer by a physiotherapist of relaxation sessions may be warmly accepted because often there has been nobody available to teach the techniques. (Relaxation is also discussed in Chapter 7.)

Physical Assessment

The physiotherapist provides a general physical assessment

service for those whose physical problems may cause difficulties on return to the community. The aim of acute in-patient mental illness units is to assess patients and initiate treatment quickly so that the patient can return home to continue treatment. Physical disability must not be allowed to become a barrier to a patient's return to the community.

Case History (3.2)

Mrs. *B* was a 62-year-old retired teacher. She had suffered from asthma throughout her life and was taking steroid drug therapy as a result of which she was overweight, moon-faced and had osteoporosis. Mrs. *B* had saved up her steroid drugs over a long period and was regularly taking a far higher dose than her medical practitioner had prescribed. Mrs. *B* began to suffer from the effects of a steroid induced psychosis (an acute confusional state). She became suspicious and fearful of others. One day from her flat on the first floor she saw her son arrive to visit her. As she heard him come up the stairs she thought he was coming to kill her. Mrs. *B* jumped from the window to escape and sustained crush fractures of two thoracic vertebrae and a fractured tibia and fibula.

She was admitted to the sick bay of the psychiatric hospital. The orthopaedic surgeon from the general hospital discussed physical management with the physiotherapist and Mrs. *B* was quickly mobilised and her drugs adjusted. A case conference was called and the physiotherapist met the community psychiatric nurse who would be visiting Mrs. *B* each day. The nurse, Mrs. *B* and the physiotherapist were able to discuss how to overcome the physical problems that Mrs. *B* might encounter on returning to the flat with her leg in plaster and on elbow crutches, and in particular, climbing the steep steps up to the flat safely.

Common Acute Mental Disorders and Physiotherapy

There follow brief descriptions of the main acute mental disorders which a physiotherapist encounters and the way in which physiotherapy may be involved. These patients are often very disturbed and confused. Patience and understanding are essential on the part of the physiotherapist who should fully acquaint herself with the psychiatric history of the patient before seeing him, and plan any treatment in conjunction with the ward team. The advice of the ward team should be sought if difficulty is encountered in establishing a rapport with a patient. The physiotherapist must make regular reports to the ward team on patient progress in order to integrate treatment. This is crucial to the treatment of all patients and cannot be overemphasised, especially as a physiotherapist who is not necessarily a continuous member of a team could seriously disrupt a treatment programme, even with the best of intentions, if not fully in touch with the ward team about a specific case.

Depression

The various types of depression account for 20% of admissions to psychiatric hospitals in England.[1] Only the most severely depressed people are admitted to hospital, the majority are treated by their own doctors at home or seek no treatment.

Various schools of thought exist on the classification of depression. Even the most severe types of depression have been shown to be associated with external circumstances so that the terms reactive and endogenous cannot always be used by some research workers. In general it is recognised that certain symptom clusters are associated with a good response to physical methods of treatment, for example ECT or antidepressant drugs. Such symptoms include:

Loss of appetite and weight
Early morning wakening
Abnormal guilt
Slowness of thought, speech and actions
Poor concentration
Psychotic phenomena such as delusions of which the content is gloomy.

Other symptom clusters are not associated with a good outcome after medication. These include:

Difficulty in getting off to sleep
A tendency to blame others
A feeling of unhappiness which, though exaggerated, is perhaps understandable given the person's circumstances.

When biological symptoms such as weight loss and early morning wakening are prominent then the depression may be termed *biological depression*. When psychotic features are present it may be termed *psychotic depression*.

These two types of depression are often associated with *mania* at other times in a patient's life and also with a family history of depressive disorder. Depression associated with the second cluster of symptoms may be most effectively treated by psychotherapy but it should be noted that in all types of depression it is not always the case that the treatment is successful.

Physical Problems Associated with Depression

The majority of depressed patients in an acute unit will not encounter the physiotherapist for direct treatment. These patients will however feature largely in any general group work and can be helped. It must be strongly emphasised that the severely depressed need a very gentle approach and an over hearty physiotherapist could be disastrous. In group work allowances must be made for this. As a patient's depression lifts, exercise can become more positive and beneficial and is regarded by some as an effective alternative to drug therapy.

The effects of general debility and poor posture of many depressives can be countered by the inclusion of specific postural exercises and general strengthening exercises in a ward group. The negative effects of the drugs taken by patients will hamper the progress of a group. Of these negative effects sedation, blurred vision and postural hypotension are most common. Excessive weight gain may restrict mobility in patients taking monoamine oxidase inhibitors (MAOI drugs).

Specific Physiotherapy

Chest Infection

Chest infections are common in elderly, depressed persons and smokers. Treatment in preparation for, and during, a course of ECT is sometimes required in order to enable a general anaesthetic to be given. A chest infection can also ensue after a suicide attempt if the patient has been unconscious for some time, or inhaled vomit.

Case History (3.3)

Mrs. C was 52 years old and suffered from severe depression. She was emaciated from malnutrition and had contracted pneumonia with a partial collapse of one lung. The psychiatrist had decided that a course of ECT was the treatment of choice, however the anaesthetist could not give an anaesthetic because of the chest condition. The physiotherapist instituted an intensive course of postural drainage and breathing exercises. Mrs. C was walked through the grounds to the physiotherapy department as part of the treatment to improve her physical condition. Ten days later the lung had fully expanded and prophylactic physiotherapy was given throughout the course of ECT. The treatment was successful and the patient was taken away on holiday by her husband.

Severe Debility

A major programme to rehabilitate a severely undernourished, depressed patient will sometimes be necessary. Patients admitted with severe debility are usually elderly and undernourished. Initially one should always keep the work well within the patients capabilities, over-enthusiasm could swamp what little desire the patient has to improve. For younger patients a very gently graded circuit can be the answer.

Case History (3.4)

Mr. D was 56 years old and had suffered a stroke five years ago. He had a residual left-sided hemiplegia with a painful spastic hand. Mr. D was living an isolated life with his dominant wife. He became increasingly depressed and refused to eat. Eventually his debilitation resulted in his admission to the general hospital where he suffered a cardiac arrest. Mr. *D* was revived, and following his discharge from the intensive care unit, was admitted to the sick bay of the psychiatric hospital. The nurses gently coaxed him into eating a little and the physiotherapists tried to mobilise him. Mr. *D* was extremely frail, exhausted quickly and was unwilling to try and help himself. Mr *D* had ceased to attempt to place his left arm in an antispasm pattern and held it in the typical synergic pattern of tonic contraction. The physiotherapist stretched the hand, arm and shoulder manually rather than using an inflatable splint. Manual stretching afforded the maximum amount of communication through touch between the patient and therapist during this phase when Mr. *D* was withdrawn and uncommunicative. Mr. *D* experienced considerable relief of pain as his arm became freer and this close contact and relief of pain proved to be the basis for a good working relationship between patient and physiotherapist. The patient's left leg had a mild degree of extensor spasm but he could voluntarily move it into the antispasm pattern. Mr. *D*'s balance was poor and he was impeded by both frailty and his mental state. The mental health care team needed to transfer Mr. *D* to an acute psychiatric ward as a matter of urgency in order for him to receive a balanced treatment programme including group therapy and occupational therapy. In view of the erratic nature of some of the other patients on the new ward and Mr. *D*'s frailty the physiotherapist taught Mr. *D* to use a walking frame as a temporary measure until he became stronger.

Mr. *D* began to recover mentally and physically with the added stimulation on the acute unit. A sparkle of his old self came through and he began to overcome his physical and mental problems together. Mr. *D*'s timetable included daily physiotherapy. Mr. *D* revealed a strong sense of humour and was able to laugh at himself. His witty quips enlivened the department and raised the mood of other patients there. Those patients in turn encouraged him to conquer his acute fear of falling and boosted his ego by their open admiration of his fortitude. Mr. *D* began to talk more freely of the cause of his depression, his inability to get about independently in his village because he tired quickly, the neglect of his garden which he loved, and the loneliness and isolation.

The ward team came together to help Mr. *D* and his wife plan a more productive life at home.

One year later the physiotherapist was hailed from a smart new electric wheelchair as she shopped in a nearby village. It was Mr. *D* returning from a twice weekly visit to a day centre. He looked a new man, he explained that he used the wheelchair for long distance travel only. He was able to shop, go to the library and the day centre and often visited the village school at playtimes. He now had a heated greenhouse which enabled him to grow plants in comfort. In addition he and his wife were making regular evening trips to a social club in the nearby town where they could eat or drink and enjoy the organised entertainments.

Physical Handicap or Illness

If a patient is suffering from a major physical handicap such as paraplegia or a major progressive illness such as multiple sclerosis, he is particularly at risk from an episode of depression. Such patients whose ongoing physical problems are great, quickly deteriorate physically without the support of someone who understands their disability. The painful nature of spasm, the importance of positioning, surgical appliances and unavoidable incontinence are not readily understood by staff with psychiatric training. The rapport between the patient, the physiotherapist and the ward team in these cases is vital to the patients successful recovery from depression (*see* Case History 6.1).

Self Inflicted Injury

The physiotherapist may more rarely encounter a patient with self inflicted injury. The following types of injury are most likely to require physiotherapy:

Nerve and tendon damage following wrist slashing
Fractures as a result of a jump
Brain damage due to anoxia following hanging or self-poisoning, and formerly from an unsuccessful gassing attempt

Chest infections
Gun shot wounds (uncommon in the United Kingdom).

The physiotherapist is primarily treating the body but is one member of the treatment team who spends some time with the patient in a one-to-one relationship. It follows that these patients may come to talk more freely to their physiotherapist than to some others. Consequently, thoughts of suicide expressed by a patient must be reported to the ward team. The physiotherapist may have been told something which others have not. In addition the physiotherapist always touches the patient during treatment, and this communication through touch is again emphasised at this stage as it can be an important link towards communication through speech.

Case History (3.5)

Mrs. *E* was a 32-year-old teacher who had had her first child three months ago. Both parents had desperately wanted a child, but because of her age Mrs. *E* had given up a well established career when she became pregnant. After the birth and taking the baby home Mrs. *E* became increasingly depressed, she felt unable to relate to her baby emotionally in any way and began to neglect her. Mrs. *E* took an overdose of salicylates and was admitted to an acute psychiatric unit under a Section Order.

It took several months of therapy involving the whole family including grandparents who were looking after the baby, before the Section Order was lifted and Mrs. *E* was making regular trips home. One evening during a ward Christmas Party Mrs. *E* went into the toilet and slashed her left wrist with a dinner knife, severing the tendons of flexor carpi radialis and flexor pollicis longus. These were sutured and the wrist immobilised. The physiotherapy department was alerted and the physiotherapist made herself known to the patient. When the plaster was removed from the wrist Mrs. *E* came to the department to mobilise the hand. The physiotherapist did not probe into the events surrounding the accident. Mrs. *E* was clearly embarrassed by the renewed Section Order and hated being escorted by the physiotherapy helper to the department and back. The helper tried to counteract this by utilising the trip out, enabling Mrs. *E* to call in at the hospital shop on the way to the department, or by taking a short walk through the gardens.

One day Mrs. *E* felt sufficiently at ease with the physiotherapist to confide in her. She told of her inability to love the baby and the desperate fears that she never would and that one day, she might harm the baby. The physiotherapist spoke to the ward team about what had been said and was encouraged by their support. They said that Mrs. *E* was normally very reserved and it was good that she felt able to confide.

Mrs. *E* stayed as a voluntary patient for some time after her wrist was better and subsequently went home with considerable back-up from the community services.

Manic Depressive Illness

Patients in a manic phase of a depressive illness are accident prone due to their hyperactivity and inability to concentrate. Minor injury such as bruising is common and occasionally a major injury such as a fracture is sustained. These patients may regularly rip off bandages and plasters and ignore advice during this acute mania. As a result of this lack of cooperation it is possible that there will be a final deformity or lack of function which might otherwise have been prevented.

Case History (3.6)

Mr. *F*, aged 20, crashed his motorbike. He fractured his right patella and his right radius and ulna at the wrist. The patella was excised and both knee and wrist were immobilised in plaster. Mr *F* discharged himself from hospital and soaked off the plasters in the bath at home.

Two months later Mr. *F* crashed his bike again and coincidentally fractured his left patella which was also excised. Once again he removed his leg plaster. Mr. *F* became hyperactive and unmanageable at home and two months after the second injury he was admitted to the acute ward of a psychiatric hospital under a section of the Mental Health Act.

Mr. *F* was calmed with drugs but the soporific effect of the drugs combined with his weak knees meant that he was always falling down. The physiotherapist was asked to assess Mr. *F*'s physical problems.

Mr. *F* walked by throwing his knees into hyperextension and locking the knees to take his weight. He had an 80° quadriceps lag on one leg and a 60° lag on the other. In addition, the wrist fracture was ununited and the wrist swollen and tender.

Mr. *F*'s powers of concentration were minimal, he would perform an exercise half heartedly a few times and stop. He never performed any exercise to its full range unless the physiotherapist monitored every movement personally. Often Mr. *F* fell asleep after a few minutes as a result of his drug therapy. Nevertheless Mr. *F* began to gain considerably more control over his legs. One day while the physiotherapist was escorting him back to the ward he walked off in the wrong direction at remarkable speed saying he was going home to get some clean clothes. The physiotherapist did not remonstrate but ran straight to the ward and the police brought Mr. *F* back in cheerful mood some hours later. After this Mr. *F*'s Section Order was rescinded and he became calmer.

A case conference was held and it was decided that as a result of the physiotherapist's report on Mr. *F*'s poor physical condition and with Mr. *F*'s agreement a place should be sought for him in a residential rehabilitation unit for a short period as soon as his mental state allowed.

Anxiety States

Anxiety states may exist on their own or very commonly be combined with another psychiatric disorder such as depression. An overwhelming sense of fear and worry, the inability to cope with simple tasks, poor concentration and agitation are some of the psychological symptoms.

Physical Symptoms

Patients with anxiety states have many physical symptoms resulting from overactivity of the autonomic nervous system. The patients then worry about these physical symptoms thereby making them worse. Palpitations, dry mouth, intestinal and bladder problems, also head, back and neck ache are common. In addition hyperventilation produces many symptoms such as dizziness, paraesthesia or blackouts. A great deal of importance is attached to these symptoms by the patient who sees them as the primary problem. These physical symptoms also lead to a fear on the patient's part that he may be going to die or to have a heart attack or some other serious physical illness.

Treatment

Treatment of anxiety neurosis by tranquillisers alone is all too common. Patients quickly become dependent on these drugs which are habit forming and withdrawal symptoms are experienced when reducing the dose. However, the use of drugs may be necessary in the short term, enabling the patient to sleep, and to think more clearly. Psychological treatment to help the patient understand the root of the problem and the origin of the physical symptoms, coupled with a course of relaxation training are probably the treatments of choice. Nevertheless some anxiety states do become chronic.

Physiotherapy in Anxiety States

Physical Assessment

The physiotherapist may be asked to give a complete physical assessment of the patient. The patient may have had much physical treatment for his symptoms either from other physiotherapists or from some of the various alternative therapists. Sometimes the cause of pain may be due to a long-term postural defect accentuated by spasm due to tension. The original cause of the anxiety may be lost way back in a patient's life and the patient is left with a physical habit such as hyperventilation or hunched shoulders which can be corrected.

The concise physical assessment, particularly for those who have had much physical treatment is a great help to those about to give psychological help. If the physical symptoms are paramount in the patient's mind, then the patient must be able to accept a logical explanation of them combined with an understanding of the autonomic mechanism which triggers off the symptoms.

Relaxation Therapy (*see* Chapter 7)

Relaxation therapy is important in helping to alleviate the symptoms of anxiety. The patient should be taught a method of relaxation to suit him and how to apply it both as a method of resting and more urgently, in problem situations.

Planning

After receiving help for an anxiety state a patient may expect to be able to cope with the busy routine of home and work where many of the problems which precipitated the illness may still be unsolved. This unrealistic expectation combined with attempts to reduce drug dosage renders the patient at risk in situations where he is unable to cope and the old anxiety symptoms will be experienced again. The physiotherapist can help by giving practical advice on planning the physical day. Initially a routine is based on essential tasks only, which is easily achieved, so that the patient feels pleased with what has been done rather than harassed because of what is left undone. Gradually more tasks can then be introduced. Close liaison with the key therapist in the patient's treatment is essential.

The simplest ideas such as carrying shopping in two smaller bags rather than one heavy one are often overlooked. Advice on lifting, especially where there are demanding young children in the house is also useful.

Case History (3.7)

Mrs. *G* was 34 years old, married with sons of eight and two years. Both children had been born by artificial insemination. Mrs. *G* was increasingly obsessed by thoughts that she felt unclean because of the artificial insemination. She found the younger child hard to cope with, especially if he had tantrums, and the older child was very hyperactive and disobedient taking advantage of her weaknesses.

Mrs. G had always been of an anxious disposition and had been subject to attacks of hyperventilation and blackouts since before the children were born. She developed a severe low backache which prevented her bending down to lift the younger child or change his nappy. She was admitted to an acute psychiatric ward totally unable to cope with life at home.

The psychiatric team asked the physiotherapist to assess Mrs. G's physical problems and come to a meeting to discuss whether physiotherapy might help in conjunction with the group and family therapy she would have to help solve problems.

The physiotherapist planned a treatment scheme as part of the patient's individual programme. Initially Mrs. G was taught how to recognise the onset of a hyperventilation attack. Relaxation in different positions was taught and breathing exercises to calm and control her breathing. Mrs. G found this extremely valuable and responded well to advice.

Mrs. G's posture was poor, she stooped with bowed head and hunched shoulders. She held her trunk rigid unwilling to bend or twist saying it hurt. A short relaxation session at the start of each treatment helped her to calm her mind and body. She then progressed to back mobility exercises with the emphasis on free movement. At a later stage, together with other patients in the department, some free work to music was introduced and much enjoyed.

Mrs. G continued to insist she could not lift her child, even though her backache was much improved. Lifting instruction was instituted reinforcing her ability to turn and bend and pick up inanimate objects. When Mrs. G started to go home for short periods a progressive daily plan was worked out as described in the section on planning (*see* p. 27). Initially there were problems such as trying to catch-up on household chores late in the evening instead of relaxing, but Mrs. G gradually began to cope. The community psychiatric services offered strong support and Mrs. G was also able to enjoy the daytime company and activity of a local authority keep fit class which provided crêche facilities.

Phobias

A phobia is a type of anxiety characterised by fear in particular situations. Some phobias may be extremely specific such as phobias of snakes, but other phobias are more general such as agoraphobia. Patients with these difficulties are usually treated in extramural services.

Types of Phobia

Simple Phobia

Simple phobia is an irrational fear of one specific thing, for example, birds, spiders, darkness or heights. These are the least common phobias.

Social Phobias

Social phobias are fears of situations involving other people such as a fear of blushing or an inability to eat in a restaurant for fear of vomiting. It is feared that these events could then induce ridicule or criticism from others.

Agoraphobia

This is a common phobia. A major panic attack, classically in a supermarket queue initiates a fear of similar attacks in crowded situations. The patient gradually becomes housebound with an excessive emotional hold on her family on whom she depends totally for her daily needs. Life for all becomes very restricted and family relationships fraught.

Treatment

Tranquillising drugs may be used in the short term but are less likely to be the treatment chosen in the long term rather than behavioural therapy.

Patients are taught to face their fears (on a graduated basis) and how to combat the panic reactions which result. The control of tension by relaxation, biofeedback or other method is taught. The appropriate anxiety provoking situation is then gradually introduced with the patient using the tension control technique to prevent panic.

Physiotherapy

Psychologists and nurse therapists trained in behavioural therapy usually treat phobias. However, in some cases the physiotherapist is asked to train the patient in a suitable relaxation technique and how to apply it appropriately.

Hysteria

The diagnosis of hysteria as a specific condition is difficult. Up to 33% of patients diagnosed as having a hysterical condition in one survey were subsequently proved to have an organic cause for their symptoms.[2] The patient may seem surprisingly unconcerned about quite a severe disability produced by hysterical symptoms. This is termed *'la belle indifférence'*.

Conversion Hysteria

Conversion hysteria, though rare, is the form most likely to be encountered by the physiotherapist as it can often involve neurological symptoms such as muscular weakness, paralysis or pain. Hysterical fits, vomiting and many other unexplained physical symptoms may be unconsciously produced. A patient who appears to have been cured of one symptom such as backache, subsequently presents with a new symptom if the real root of the problem is not resolved.

Other Forms of Hysteria

Occasionally episodes of mass hysteria are encountered such as a whole class of school children fainting and being admitted to hospital. The label hysterical is all too often applied to people. Women are more likely to be labelled as hysterical rather than men.

Physiotherapy in Conversion Hysteria

In the rare cases where physiotherapy is indicated, the physiotherapist working in the field of mental health who is most qualified to cope with a hysterical patient, is unfortunately usually the last of a series of physiotherapists to encounter this patient. The patient may have had a great deal of treatment for the physical symptoms which will have been of no benefit since the underlying causes of the condition were psychological.

Assessment

The physiotherapist may be asked to assess the patient physically. The physiotherapist should be aware that inconsistencies such as the ability to remain continent in a rare case of hysterical paraplegia are to be expected. Indeed there may be little value in a formal physical assessment of such a patient. The main problem is to remember that at all times symptoms produced by the patient are unconscious. The physiotherapist should put aside any feelings of being misled by the patient. The patient is equally misled.

Waiting

While the basic psychological problems are being resolved the physiotherapist is unlikely to be needed. A point of contact between the patient and the physiotherapist can be maintained through the ward movement group. A patient with gross disablement will need some general advice on how to cope with the disability while it lasts but specific physical treatment will not help the patient's recovery.

Rehabilitation

Once a patient starts to resolve the problems underlying the hysteria, the physical symptoms may disappear dramatically and rapidly. If however, a particular physical situation has been prolonged, disuse atrophy may result. In such a case a treatment scheme can be quickly instituted and recovery will probably be speedily achieved.

Case History (3.8)

Miss *H* was admitted to an acute psychiatric ward under a Section Order. She was 31 and wheelchair-bound with hysterical paraplegia. Miss *H*'s complaint originally presented with backache prior to her nursing final examinations. She had never taken her finals, and from then on had become increasingly disturbed. Following a car accident Miss *H* had sustained a fractured left tibial malleolus which had been pinned; since then she had been unable to walk or to move her legs. Miss *H* mutilated herself continually, slashing her wrists and cutting the flesh of her forearms and thighs with anything sharp. She also attempted to set fire to herself, the ward, or her belongings if she was allowed matches. Miss *H* had recently attended a rehabilitation centre where physical treatment had been of no benefit.

The consultant psychiatrist asked the physiotherapist to assess Miss *H*'s physical capabilities and give the rest of the ward team guidelines on the temporary care of the patient's paraplegia. Cases of hysterical paralyses rarely follow a logical anatomical pattern because they do not have a physical cause. In long sitting, Miss *H* held her legs with feet vertical when flail limbs might have been expected to roll into inversion or eversion; also Miss *H* was continent of urine and faeces. The physiotherapist noted this without comment, accepting that the extent of the paralysis was entirely unconscious. However the wasting of the lower limb muscles and the injured ankle which had never borne weight since the accident alerted the physiotherapist to the fact that she would be needed to help with this problem when the time came.

Miss *H* seemed unconcerned by her paralysis and it took three months of frustrating work by the ward team before the patient began to stop mutilating herself and became less disturbed. During this time the physiotherapist only saw Miss *H* during the course of her other work on the ward, but she always made a point of speaking to her.

Miss *H* made friends with another patient and they decided to live together when they left hospital. The friend was discharged, and soon after Miss *H* asked to come to the physiotherapy department and try to walk. Miss *H* was surprised by her weakness and the pinned ankle was so painful when she put her weight on it that it was necessary to ice the ankle prior to exercise. It took Miss *H* four weeks to get herself on her feet and she left hospital as soon as she had progressed from using elbow crutches to using sticks.

Anorexia Nervosa

Anorexia nervosa is a disorder suffered mainly by adolescent young women. In this condition the young woman has a distorted perception of her body image and perceives herself as grossly fat and unattractive. The young woman then deliberately restricts her diet to the point of starvation and even death still maintaining the gross image of herself. Sometimes the patient resorts to binge eating and vomiting (bulimia), many are physical fitness fanatics determined to work off every last centimetre of spare fat.

The original cause of the anorexia is often tied up in complicated family relationships and the core of the problem may be an unsatisfactory relationship with a dominant mother combined with fears about reaching physical maturity and social pressures from peer groups or others about being overweight.

Treatment is initially by achieving weight gain to a safe level which is sometimes followed by physiotherapy.

Physiotherapy and Anorexia Nervosa

There are two opposing schools of thought among those who manage the treatment of anorexia nervosa with regard to physiotherapy: There are those who say physiotherapy is contraindicated and believe that, because anorexics are often intent on exercising to lose weight, any form of physical activity if stressed will reinforce the need to exercise and reduce weight. Thus physiotherapists should avoid contact with anorexic patients.

A second school of thought believes that as the anorexic gains weight she needs to re-educate her false perceptions of body image. Also if she regains weight without any attention to musculature she will indeed look flabby and puffed out. In this instance the physiotherapist may be asked to work with the patient in the field of body awareness and perception. This can be done in conjunction with any psychotherapy being received.

The aims would be to work towards the recognition of

the feel and look of the normal healthy body. Creative movement involving spatial awareness and the feel of the body can be introduced. A long mirror and the use of touch can help reinforce a correct body image. The patient should be helped to appreciate the difference between healthy physical activity and extreme physical fanaticism.

Schizophrenia

Schizophrenia is a common illness in all cultures. In the western world about 1% of adults are diagnosed as schizophrenic at some time in their lives. Acute schizophrenia is a young person's illness occurring in the 20–39 age group mainly, with a peak age range of 25–30 years. More men than women are affected.

Schizophrenia is diagnosed in terms of symptoms which indicate an inability on the part of the patient to differentiate between his inner self in his own mind and the world around him.

Schizophrenia may present acutely or insidiously. Those with an insidious onset and who are younger and with poor emotional responses are more likely to have a chronic or relapsing course of their illness, but of all schizophrenics, up to three-quarters relapse after recovering from their first illness.

Schizophrenia is a major management problem for the mental health care team. The symptoms may be divided into positive symptoms and negative symptoms.

Positive Symptoms

Acute, florid schizophrenic episodes are diagnosed by positive symptoms, these include:

Delusions of Thought Interference

Thoughts are inserted into or taken out of the mind. Thoughts may also be broadcast and therefore known to others. Delusions are false, fixed beliefs held by the patient despite evidence to the contrary.

Auditory Hallucinations

Voices continually repeat or anticipate thoughts in the patient's mind. Voices may comment on private thoughts or discuss the patient in the third person as 'he'. For the patient, the perception of these voices is exactly the same as the perception of a real conversation.

Delusions of Control

A delusional feeling that some external force is controlling the emotions or movements, and thus the schizophrenic is often compelled to perform an irrational act.

Delusions of Perception

Everyday occurrences such as a 'phone ringing or another person's cough may be perceived as having special, often sinister meaning for the patient.

Negative Symptoms

These symptoms include:

Poverty of Speech
Poverty of Movement
Lack of Motivation
Flatness of Effect or Emotion
Social Withdrawal

Treatment of Schizophrenia

Recurrent schizophrenia cannot be cured but treatment has improved so that the majority of sufferers no longer crowd the wards of psychiatric hospitals.

When an acute attack occurs treatment is usually started by admission to hospital. While the acute symptoms are curbed by medication, the patient and his family are assessed so that decisions can be made regarding the future. The counselling of the family is most important, and some think the family's reaction to the illness is crucial. Some research suggests that in cases where the family continually interreact over-emotionally when the patient is at home then the patient is more likely to relapse.

Since the introduction of depot injections of phenothiazine the effects of which last for up to one month, management of schizophrenia in the community is easier. In the days when the patient had to take tablets regularly there was no guarantee that he would do so, and relapses into an acute state were unexpected and uncontrollable if the patient lived outside an institution. A patient who does not turn up to a regular injection clinic is quickly identified as 'at risk' and the case is followed up by the community psychiatric nurse. Patients with chronic schizophrenia may need drug therapy throughout their lifetime.

Physiotherapy Involvement with Schizophrenia

Acute Schizophrenia

The patient admitted during an acute attack of schizophrenia is very disturbed. Even when drug therapy is established he may be unable to relate to the simplest routines of ward life. The schizophrenic with no physical problems is unlikely to meet the physiotherapist except in a general movement session. The nursing staff may advise against this if the patient is suffering strong delusions of control. It is doubtful whether joining in a movement group is of benefit in acute schizophrenia. Although it is postulated by some physiotherapists that simple specific movement work may help the schizophrenic to differentiate between reality and delusions, no research has been produced to support this. Schizophrenics are often unable to tolerate extraneous noise because of the confused input of their hallucinations. Music therefore, or noise from other patients, may impede successful involvement in a group. Group movement work is much more useful with chronic schizophrenic patients (*see* Chapter 4).

Trauma

The physiotherapist will need to be directly involved if the acute schizophrenic episode has resulted in trauma. Schizophrenics have a higher rate of parasuicide and suicide than the general population, often as a result of delusions of control.

A typical sequence of events might be, hearing footsteps on the stairs, voices saying 'Let's go and murder the silly old fool'; 'But he'll probably jump out of the window before we get there'; 'Look, he's going over to the window, just going to jump out'; 'Silly old fool'. The delusion is so strong that the schizophrenic jumps out of a window and incurs fractures.

Initially the patient will be disturbed and probably sedated. The physiotherapist is in a difficult position, she must get the patient moving but must not allow herself to be confused with the delusions of control which have just precipitated the accident. If this happened it could cause withdrawal, mistrust and aggression in the patient. The physiotherapist's approach should be informal, relaxed and quietly friendly without intrusion into mental problems or the cause of the accident. If a patient refuses treatment, the physiotherapist should go away and come back later, working at being accepted by the patient as someone he sees regularly, can trust, and who is seen to be on good terms with others on the ward. Complete flexibility on the part of the physiotherapist is important. The nursing staff may be able to advise on the best time of day to institute treatment as there may be some regular times when the patient is less disturbed.

Exercise routines should be very basic and simple, always starting with work which is easy and enjoyed. The patient himself may be more cooperative if he chooses the starting work, new work can be attempted as the patient relaxes. Extraneous noise such as a patient shouting in another part of the department or a radio playing can be intolerable and prevent concentration.

If a patient has a potential for violence, crutches or sticks could be used as a weapon. A walking frame may seem incongruous for a younger person but it is far less easy to hit out with. Some schizophrenics abhor artificial aids and refuse to use walking aids and take off bandages or splints. These patients are at risk of permanent deformity or malfunction and where the physiotherapist is worried that this may happen, she should alert the ward team as an adjustment of drugs may be indicated for the required physiotherapy to be carried out.

A patient who has a good relationship with the physiotherapist will find that the simple exercise routines to heal a tangible injury will help him to distinguish physical reality from delusions. In order to reinforce this the physiotherapist should use touch as an aid to communication using firm, but not restricting, holds on injured limbs and asking the patient to feel the hold on them and telling him when letting go.

Delusions and hallucinations are often associated by the patient with radios, televisions and other electrical apparatus. Such apparatus in the physiotherapy department may be regarded with grave suspicion and should not be used in the treatment of acutely ill schizophrenic patients. If possible it is best kept out of sight.

The physical side-effects of the neuroleptic drugs being administered can hinder the physical rehabilitation of a schizophrenic patient (*see* Chapter 6).

Case History (3.9)

Miss *I* was 26 years old and suffering from schizophrenia. She had dropped out of university at the age of 20. From then on she took a series of clerical jobs each of which was less demanding than the previous one. Miss *I* moved about the country from job to job, rejecting offers of help from her parents and finally stopped working entirely. She was living alone in a bed sitter when she felt compelled to jump through her first floor window.

Miss *I* landed upright on both legs and sustained bilateral fractured calcanei. She was admitted to the sick bay of the psychiatric hospital to be nursed, her legs were non-weight bearing for nine weeks. The physiotherapist began the appropriate mobilisation immediately. Miss *I* was very drowsy and incoherent initially and the drug therapy contributed to this. She was quite amenable to the physiotherapist visiting her but claimed she was far too tired to do anything about moving of her own accord. The physiotherapist showed the nursing staff the basic movements that Miss *I* was to do regularly and they also encouraged these to help combat the patient's characteristic lack of drive. Miss *I* remained very vague about herself and the physiotherapist was careful not to probe. As the patient improved she became less sleepy and more communicative. She did not complain of much pain and seemed uninterested in future developments.

As soon as the physiotherapists were able to teach Miss *I* to walk safely on crutches she was transferred to an acute ward. In the sick bay she had looked fit and well cared for. In the acute ward she had to do much more for herself. Miss *I*'s personal appearance deteriorated, she could not be bothered to wash properly and looked a mess. Exercising independently was also too much and at a team meeting the physiotherapist expressed the opinion that while ideally a short period at a rehabilitation centre should be considered, in practise Miss *I* would not cope with the demanding atmosphere.

Miss *I* returned to her parents' home in a different health district and arrangements were made for local psychiatric and orthopaedic services to take over her management.

Chronic Schizophrenia

It is probably the case that most patients admitted to acute units with schizophrenia are readmissions. Physiotherapy involvement with schizophrenic patients in long term care is discussed in Chapter 4.

References

1. Department of Health and Social Security (1975). *In Patient Statistics from the Mental Health Inquiry for England.* (Statistical Research Report series no. 20.) London: HMSO.
2. Slater E. (1965). Diagnosis of hysteria. *British Medical Journal.* **1**: 1395.

Further Reading

Hackett T. P., Cassem N. H., eds (1978). *Handbook of General Hospital Psychiatry*. St Louis, USA: CV Mosby Co.

Berne E. (1964). *Games People Play*. Harmondsworth: Penguin Books.

Stanway A. (1981). *Overcoming Depression*. London: Hamlyn Paperbacks.

Mitchell R. (1982). *Phobias*. Harmondsworth: Penguin Books.

Mitchell A. R. K. (1975). *Schizophrenia – What It Means*. London: Teach Yourself Books.

4

Chronic Mental Illness

There is an increasing range of facilities for those who are chronically mentally ill. Fewer patients now spend their lives in Victorian mental hospitals. Specialised units exist for the rehabilitation of schizophrenics and other units for long-term psychotherapy. There are also specialised units for the rehabilitation of those with organic brain disease. In general chronically mentally ill patients fall into the following main groups. Those with:

Chronic forms of neuroses
Major psychoses, principally schizophrenia
Organic conditions, for example, head injury, epilepsy, Huntington's chorea
Personality disorders.

Nowadays units for the care of the chronically mentally ill would be described as practising social therapy. The aim of these units is to help their members to lead purposeful, active, free and responsible lives[1] under the guidance of psychiatrists and the rest of the mental health care team. Two professions have come to the fore in the practice of social therapy, notably the psychiatric nurse who is the mainstay of support for the patient, and the occupational therapist who organises productive work for those needing sheltered workshop facilities and teaches activities for independent daily living and purposeful recreation. Other professions such as psychologists, art and music therapists have strong supporting roles.

Currently patients who have been in hospital wards for many years are being prepared for life in the community. All professions involved in their care are actively working towards this goal. Some professions are having to reappraise their work with a view to being more involved in the community care of the mentally ill and discover how they can best utilise their skills in that context. This applies to any of the strongly hospital based therapies such as physiotherapy, and the role of the physiotherapist in the community care of the mentally ill will have to be carefully evaluated.

The majority of the chronically mentally ill will be on permanent drug therapy which needs constant monitoring by their doctors and some patients suffer unpleasant side-effects from the drugs (*see* Chapter 6).

Social Therapy in a Psychiatric Hospital

The long-stay hospital ward in an old Victorian hospital is likely to remain for some years, although the ultimate goal is to close these units. Young, chronically mentally ill people are rarely admitted to these units any more but are looked after by the community services. A group of ageing patients remain, many of them schizophrenic, who were placed in custodial care long before modern improvements in treatments and drug therapy. The long-stay wards are their home and may have been so since before the Second World War. These people will have memories of the restrictions of locked wards, sedation and physical restraint. Although much has been done to humanise surroundings it is difficult to make a small room, designed to confine a patient, into an attractive bedroom.

Toilet facilities may still be very basic and provide inadequate privacy for the sexes. Dormitories have been decorated attractively and individual furniture provided but the high ceilings and windows and narrow staircases are still there. The physical conditions in which the chronically mentally ill are obliged to live are a matter of great concern to those involved in their care.

Within the hospital, as an aid to ultimate independence, there may be various grades of accommodation. Bedsitters or housing units in the grounds may be used by people living totally independently, learning to run a home of their own and manage on a budget, or waiting for accommodation in the community. Certain wards may be run on a hostel basis. The hospital provides accommodation and food and the ward residents run the ward between themselves agreeing on work rotas and general policies to enable a satisfactory communal life. A member of staff will be available in the daytime to help solve problems but there is no nurse permanently on the ward at night. Other wards may be run on similar lines but night cover may be provided.

Every hospital needs its heavy dependency wards for the more mentally infirm. These wards have a high staff patient ratio, thus if a patient has a violent outburst more nurses are available. Experienced nurses are adept at calming down a patient who is being aggressive, usually by talking the problem through. As soon as it is practical a group of those staff and patients involved in the incident will form and a chance to vent feelings is given to try to resolve the problem. Such outbursts are comparatively rare and often avoidable. There is far less aggression between male patients on mixed sex wards and the only reason why some hospitals have all female wards is that there are more women patients than men.

In addition the ageing of many long-stay patients has resulted in wards being adapted to the failing ability and mobility of the residents. On these wards the physiotherapist is increasingly in demand.

The pattern of the day mapped out for patients will centre around independence. Dressing, care of possessions, cleanliness, care of surroundings and purposeful occupation are major goals. The most active may spend the day working in a sheltered workshop. The less able will have other opportunities offered to them such as self expression through art and music therapy, daily living activities such as cooking, managing money, good grooming, physical recreation and drama work. Most wards are devoid of people except at meal times. Individual patients may go out shopping or on business with or without an accompanying nurse. Staff and patients have regular meeting times when they come together to review the ongoing situation.

Day Centres and Community Work

As the numbers of psychiatric hospitals are reduced so day centres are being set up to provide the activities which were formerly provided by the hospital. Patients leaving the hospitals may live in a variety of types of accommodation including hostels and houses funded by health authorities or local authorities or managed by voluntary organisations. Others may have their own homes or be able to live with their families supported by community psychiatric staff. Small units called group homes are increasingly favoured. Such a home is frequently a large house in which a number of people live together with communal sitting and catering facilities. The group needs to be able to work together to organise the fair share of housework and catering and will meet regularly as a group together with a member of the psychiatric team to discuss this. Unfortunately increasing numbers of chronically mentally ill people find themselves placed in lonely seaside boarding houses where they have little to do and no day centre facilities are provided. In areas where this has occurred community care has fallen far short of the ideal.

While all the physical problems of patients in hospital, which are discussed in the rest of this chapter, will remain with the patient when he moves into the community, the role of the physiotherapist and her access to mentally ill patients in the community is as yet undefined. It is certain that physiotherapists working in the community will come into increasing contact with the mentally ill and those who have no knowledge or experience of the mentally ill will be obliged to educate themselves in the subject. Some authorities have already decided that a physiotherapist should be appointed with a specific brief for the care of the mentally ill in the community. This is an exciting new prospect, for it means that the physiotherapist can set up a scheme for physical care without being bound by former traditions and practices.

The setting up of physical activity groups and relaxation courses at day centres will enable the physiotherapist to get to know the patients. Physical disability can then be both prevented or treated early which will combat some of the severe problems which can be otherwise encountered. In addition the physiotherapist who knows the patients and their histories can advise other physiotherapists, both in the community and in general hospital departments, on the best methods of approach for particular patients and their illnesses. The lack of ability to communicate, particularly among the schizophrenic population, does mean that some physical problems can become quite severe before they are noticed by staff who are trained in mental health care but not in physical care. The physiotherapist working in mental health can fill this gap and act as a troubleshooter for physical problems. This is one area of health care where the institution of a fitness programme could readily be incorporated with lasting effect.

The importance of the ideals and ideas set out in the preceding paragraphs in regard to the role of the physiotherapist in modern psychiatric practice should be emphasised at this point. If community care is to provide a good quality of life for the mentally ill then professionals such as physiotherapists should be involved from the outset of a new project.

However the physiotherapist will need to consider carefully how involved she should become within the smaller community units such as hostels and group homes. Unlike a day centre which people attend for guided activity and treatment, small living units are people's private homes. Privacy is something everyone values, especially in their own home and the community team as a whole will respect this and try and reach the correct balance between giving help when needed and unwarranted intrusion into private lives. Thus no specific guidelines can be given as to which type of unit may need a physiotherapy input and this is likely to vary according to the dependency of the patients in any specific home. Undoubtedly the most important factors, where a physiotherapist has a specific brief to work with the mentally ill in the community, are that she be known to patients and the mental health care team, that they know what she has to offer and that she is accessible.

Since the entire area of community psychiatric care is still being established it is important for those physiotherapists newly appointed in this field to record and evaluate both the successes and the failures in their work. The results of this work must then be published in order to give specific guidance to future planners on the benefits or otherwise, of a physiotherapy input into community psychiatry.

The Therapeutic Community

The concept of the therapeutic community was developed by Maxwell Jones as a result of his work with psychologically damaged soldiers towards the end of the Second World War. In the 1950s and 1960s a few hospitals developed their chronic wards along the lines of the therapeutic community concept. This concept was intensely emotionally demanding on all involved. Staff and patients worked together in small and large groups, discussing, arguing, criticising and reassessing themselves and others and their role in the community. They analysed the way in which the community was running itself and attempted to help each other in solving individual problems.

It was in this setting that staff began to abandon the use of the formal uniform which it was felt created a barrier between the treater and the treated. The therapeutic community concept requires intense personal interaction and committed group involvement. This concept was a change which was completely accepted by some but only partly by many.

Physiotherapy for the Chronically Mentally Ill

The physiotherapist has three roles in the treatment of the chronically mentally ill. These are first, the maintenance of physical independence, second to supervise the provision of aids to physical independence, and third to treat specific physical problems.

The Maintenance of Physical Independence

People who live in institutions or in the community but who are insufficiently occupied may develop a stooping, listless posture and general poverty of movement. Many are heavy smokers and have chronic chest disease. Those taking long-term neuroleptic drugs suffer from the physical problems caused by the side-effects of those drugs (*see* Chapter 6). Poor communication with others is a feature of chronic mental illness and of chronic schizophrenia in particular.

General Group Work

General movement work can be provided either on the hospital ward, in a day centre or in a physiotherapy department. The work should be purposeful and fun, incorporating music, session games and competitions to stimulate body and mind. In particular, working with others in the group to enhance intercommunication is important. It should however be remembered that some think that schizophrenics do not thrive on too much communication, and advice should be sought from the ward team on whether these patients would best be left out of group work.

The physiotherapist should not have to do or think of everything and patients can be encouraged to invent their own exercises for others to copy, choose music they like and decide on the apparatus to use. The range of activities which can be considered is wide, but depends on staffing levels and budgets. A well staffed department with funds may be able to provide trips to a local sports hall or swimming pools or there may be the opportunity to offer sporting activities of varying kinds on the premises.

In a unit where historically another profession such as occupational therapists or remedial gymnasts provide a range of physical recreation activities for the more able, then the physiotherapist may be better occupied attending to those left behind rather than providing rival facilities. Indeed those left behind are the ones most at risk of losing their mobility. Gathering together those left on a ward and providing a positive and enjoyable movement session is hard work. These patients are likely to be the least responsive and most disabled. However, staff will welcome the opportunity to interest the patients and will be more available to join in and help when the able-bodied patients are out on other activities. The initial lack of response may be disheartening but it only needs one or two people to show interest and be seen to enjoy themselves before all concerned look forward to the physiotherapist's regular visits to the ward. During these movement sessions opportunities can be made to stretch knees, inspect contracted hands, walk with those who need help and keep an eye on the physical abilities of those at risk from immobility. Nursing staff can use the session to seek advice on problem patients.

Visitors to the ward can be encouraged to join in and finishing the session with a well-loved activity such as the 'Hokey-Cokey' is always appreciated. If the session comes to an end with the morning coffee round then the physiotherapist should stay and socialise for a while, obtaining patient and staff opinions on the session and seeking out ideas on further sessions and what people would like to do.

Some units have proper gymnasium facilities in which training sessions can be organised. This is especially beneficial to the younger patients who can keep records of progress in circuit work or on apparatus. In addition encouragement can be given in care of the body and general appearance. The importance of self esteem is again raised here and is amply illustrated in the following case history.

Case History (4.1)

Miss *J* was a 23 year old with severe personality problems and asthma, who had been under the care of the psychiatric department since she was in her mid-teens. Although she had come to terms with many of her problems in the last few years she engendered feelings of great hostility in many members of staff who had tried to help her during her more disturbed periods.

Miss J was living in a bedsitter room in the hospital grounds and was unemployed. She had been promised council accommodation within the next few months. Miss J began to get very fat and a severe attack of asthma and a chest infection resulted in her admission to the general hospital. When she was well enough Miss J was returned to the psychiatric hospital sick bay with a request from the chest physicians that the physiotherapist be asked to institute a fitness programme for her.

Initially her exercise tolerance was severely impaired, however she kept regular peak flow charts and with careful adjustments of her drugs by the chest physicians a steady improvement began. Miss J started to lose weight and look and feel cheerful and well. She was mentally and physically ready for a move into the community. The physiotherapist discharged Miss J expecting that she would leave the hospital within a week or so. One month later Miss J reappeared at the physiotherapy department. She had put on weight since her discharge and was complaining of pain in the right ankle. No council accommodation had been forthcoming, although promised, and she was miserable. Miss J had a history of self-inflicted injury but it had been some years since she had resorted to this. The physiotherapist and the psychiatrist were suspicious of the ankle injury, a minor sprain had been incured but the history of how it happened was ambiguous.

It was decided that the real problem was the isolation Miss J was experiencing living independently, unemployed and in a vacuum waiting for her new chance in the community. It was agreed that it would be a mistake to allow Miss J's physical well being to deteriorate in the meantime. Also Miss J's relationship with the physiotherapists was good, whereas other members of staff as previously stated, were unlikely to be sympathetic. It was agreed that Miss J would return to the physiotherapy department twice a week while she was waiting for accommodation which the medical staff would try and expedite. This she did, working independently at her circuit or joining in with others. When the new flat materialised two months later Miss J was fit and well, ready to start her new life. The physiotherapist advised Miss J to look for a local authority keep fit group to join in her new locality, where she could meet others and maintain her well being.

Relaxation (*see* Chapter 7)

Relaxation can be taught as part of a movement session or in separate sessions with the aim of reducing the many tensions experienced by the chronically mentally ill.

Aids to Independence for the Chronically Ill

The supply and maintenance of walking aids, sticks and crutches is the responsibility of the physiotherapist. Such equipment is prone to abuse owing to the erratic nature of some of those using it and a constant check needs to be kept for loose nuts and bolts and worn rubbers. The average ward, acute or chronic should have ready access to a walking frame for emergency use. On some units where there has been no physiotherapy cover for years the state and age of some aids belies description and they should be condemned and replaced.

The provision of wheelchairs is an area over which the physiotherapist needs to maintain careful control. Unless wheelchairs are ordered by the physiotherapist, who has specifically assessed a patient for his suitability for a particular chair, then problems can ensue. If wheelchairs are ordered for patients who are minimally ambulant then those patients frequently become chairbound because it is quicker for busy staff to whisk patients to the table or the toilet rather than walk slowly with them. Before long such patients are sat permanently in wheelchairs rather than being walked to easy chairs, stiff flexed joints ensue and the patient becomes wheelchair bound and immobile.

A proportion of elderly psychiatric patients who can walk a little with help are quite incapable of mastering the art of using a self-propelling wheelchair and it is this group of patients who are most at risk of permanent immobility. A unit with a number of such minimally mobile residents is best served by being supplied with a number of comfortable portering chairs suitable for use with patients when journeys out of the unit are made. For those who are minimally mobile at home a chair which can be folded to go in a car and be used for outings can be considered.

The physiotherapist may need to keep a chair with specialised attachments in reserve in the physiotherapy department. Particularly useful is a chair with elevating leg rests and a chair with a reclining back and head rest. In addition, adjustable spanners, screwdrivers and a bicycle pump are invaluable for on-the-spot adjustments to chairs as is a hand saw for shortening walking sticks.

The provision of surgical appliances is another area in which guidance may be needed, and the physiotherapist must be prepared to advise on footwear, the need for specialist aids, care of calipers and the provision of splints. Advice may be sought on the design of suitable furniture, chairs in particular, and the provision of grab rails and similar aids on wards. Each department should keep an up-to-date selection of catalogues of equipment and wheelchairs for easy reference. Referrals for specialist footwear and surgical aids can be made to local clinics.

Case History (4.2)

Mr. *K* was 66 and epileptic. He was over 1.89 m (6 ft) tall and heavy. As a teenager he had had bilateral patellectomies. He wore surgical boots for his bilateral pes cavus. Mr. *K* had lived most of his life in institutions, sent away to school as a small child he later taught at a boys' boarding school. As a young man Mr. *K* developed epilepsy and the subsequent brain damage left him less able to cope physically and mentally. Mr. *K* liked being on a heavy dependency ward, he was used to institutional life and the extreme dependency of his companions helped him to preserve his feelings of intellectual superiority and compensate for his loss of abilities.

Mr. *K* had a stroke which paralysed him down the right hand side of his body. Luckily, after a few weeks of treatment he was fully ambulant again and walking unaided. Subsequent fits and small strokes made Mr. *K* unreliable on his feet for days at a time. A borrowed wheelchair was swiftly demolished when Mr. *K*'s huge bulk crashed into it when his weak knees gave way. He refused to use a walking aid even on unreliable days, he said it slowed him up too much. He did reluctantly agree to have a wheelchair for use when his balance was so bad that he was a danger to himself and others. Consultations between the physiotherapist and the wheelchair clinic produced an old style self propelling chair which was not collapsable but much more robust than average. There was no risk of Mr. *K*'s using it unless he absolutely had to.

In addition Mr. *K*'s surgical boots had fallen to pieces. It was no problem to get a new pair, together with elastic stockings to control the oedema of the legs from which he suffered. A series of desperate appeals from the ward followed about the unsatisfactory nature of the boots. Each time the physiotherapist went to investigate Mr. *K* declared they were too tight. Each time he agreed to allow inspection the physiotherapist found he was wearing several elastic stockings and two socks on each foot and had stuffed the toes of the boots with newspapers.

It was decided that although ward policy dictated independence of dressing, and Mr. *K* was fiercely resistant to help, the nursing staff would do their best to keep a daily watch on his footwear and the physiotherapist checked him informally when she visited the ward. Mr. *K* was always more willing to accept advice from the physiotherapist rather than the nurses, and her visits enabled him to air his considerable knowledge of anatomy. He demonstrated the ongoing problems and slow deterioration faced by many on the chronic wards where patients were increasingly in need of advice on physical problems.

Specific Physical Problems

The population of an institution will suffer from time to time from any of the physical problems of the general population.

Chronic chest disease is common because so many patients smoke heavily. Neurological problems are also in greater evidence as a result of the long-term administration of neuroleptic drugs.

Trauma

Winter time is always busiest for the physiotherapist. After a sharp frost or early snowfall, wrist and ankle fractures may be expected as a result of patients slipping on the ice.

It is important that staff refer these patients to the physiotherapist immediately. The chronically mentally ill are less likely than others to remember to move fingers and shoulders prophylactically and therefore are more prone to additional complications.

Case History (4.3)

Mrs. *L*, a 60-year-old woman, was on release from a special hospital. She was profoundly depressed by the failure of a recent appeal against her compulsory detention. She lived on a hostel ward with night supervision and worked in the sheltered workshop. One morning she slipped on some black ice and sustained a left Colles' fracture. The injury was uncomplicated and the wrist was immobilised in plaster at the local accident hospital. Six weeks later the patient was taken back to the accident hospital where the plaster was removed and a tubular elastic bandage applied. The patient in her depression did not assimilate the advice given to her and the nursing helper acting as escort spoke little English.

Two weeks later a nurse telephoned the physiotherapist for advice. The elastic tubular bandage had not been removed from the hand since it had been applied but it had rolled back into a tight band round the wrist. The hand had not been washed since the original accident, the fingers and hand were grossly swollen and the skin dirty, dry and flaking. As the ward only had minimal nursing cover by nurses with psychiatric training only, they had not thought to seek advice earlier.

Fortunately it was a simple matter to soak off the dead skin, elevate the arm and start to improve function. The personal attention Mrs. *L* received in the physiotherapy department helped to break the barrier of her depression and she became motivated to use the hand functionally and soon the arm was back to normal.

The incident prompted an early meeting between the physiotherapist, senior nursing staff and junior doctors. The importance of notifying the presence of patients with all types of traumatic injury, to the physiotherapist immediately was stressed. The physiotherapists are experienced in judging who they need to follow up. Subsequently there was a considerable improvement in notifications, and physiotherapy staff also made an effort to find out about patients in plasters and bandages seen in the corridors and not recognised.

Chest Disease

Smoking exacerbates the problems of chest disease among the chronically mentally ill. Patients have little to spend their money on and face long periods of boredom in the evenings and at weekends. In the winter there is a steady stream of chest infections to treat. Psychiatrists are particularly alert to the dangers of over prescribing antibiotics in institutions where highly resistant strains of infection can so readily be bred. Physiotherapy can be used to good effect to aid the comfort and recovery of some types of chest disease and is especially useful in some cases where antibiotics are contraindicated. All group work should include some exercises aimed at improving lung function.

Aches and Pains

A constant flow of patients requires general treatments of varying kinds. Careful assessment is necessary to select those who may benefit from such treatment. Great care must be taken in using any kind of heat or electrical apparatus. Patients are unreliable even if their skin sensation is normal and may not warn the physiotherapist if it is too hot or uncomfortable and they may fiddle with apparatus when it is switched on. Flexible ice and heat packs are useful and readily understood by the patient. Warm water baths are especially good as a preliminary treatment for feet which rarely get washed.

At this point it is worth repeating the point that schizophrenic patients are likely to find electrical apparatus disturbing, because of the nature of their psychotic experiences. Basic mechanical gymnastic equipment is however often enjoyed.

Sometimes the physiotherapist needs to be very firm with other staff about inappropriate referrals. There are many long-standing physical problems among the chronically mentally ill which although preventable if they had been treated years ago cannot be improved now, and many other conditions which would never be suitable for physiotherapy.

Case History (4.4)

Miss *M* was a 57-year-old woman with manic depressive psychosis. She was thin and wirey and constantly complained of pain in her knees. Miss *M* was active and helped in the hospital launderette. Medical investigations had shown her knees to be in good condition for her age. The physiotherapist had assessed the patient and felt no help could be given. In addition the patient had aggressively indicated her unwillingness to cooperate in any form of treatment. Each time a new block of nurses or students were assigned to the ward the physiotherapist was vociferously asked why she was not treating this poor woman's painful knees. It was always difficult to convince newcomers that physiotherapy could not help this patient.

Drug Induced Physical Problems

It is among the chronically mentally ill that the lasting side-effects of some of the neuroleptic drugs are to be encountered, in particular the extrapyramidal symptoms of parkinsonism and tardive dyskinesia induced by phenothiazines and other groups of drugs. (This subject is discussed in detail in Chapter 6.)

Some Specific Chronic Mental Disorders and the Physiotherapist

Chronic Schizophrenia

The course of schizophrenia is discussed in Chapter 3. The patient with chronic schizophrenia may be suffering from negative symptoms including:

Poverty of speech
Poverty of movement
Lack of motivation
Flatness of effect and emotion
Social withdrawal.

As the patient ages he becomes less likely to lapse into acute schizophrenic states. The majority of chronic schizophrenic patients still living in long-stay units are now in their sixties and older.

No research has been published to show that physiotherapy is of any value in combatting the negative symptoms of schizophrenia.

General movement sessions are run by some physiotherapists for chronic schizophrenics and the effects of this group work need careful assessment. Free, imaginative movement, games incorporating speaking to others, expressive movements symbolising feelings, competitions, team work all help to produce a more outgoing and communicative individual, but does this necessarily apply to schizophrenics? There can be no recommended or set routines for such groups, at all times the physiotherapist must adapt her individual ideas to the needs and capabilities of the group, but above all such work needs proper evaluation.

The chronic schizophrenic patient may seem to be exceptionally tolerant of pain. This is not necessarily so, he may tolerate extremes of pain because of his inability to express emotion or communicate with others. A proportion of patients suffer from the rigidity and tremor of parkinsonism, and tardive dyskinesia which is common as a result of drug therapy.

Case History (4.5)

Mr. *N* was 59. He was a chronic schizophrenic of many years standing who lived on a minimally supervised hostel ward with no night cover and he kept himself to himself. Mr. *N* worked by day in a sheltered workshop and unobtrusively helped with his ward chores. Mr. *N*'s appearance was unkempt but he coped independently. One Friday Mr. *N* fell down the stairs but told nobody. Over the weekend he was quiet, withdrawn and more unkempt than usual. On Monday when he did not go to work the ward was contacted and the nurse in charge found Mr. *N* hidden in a corner of the coffee shop. He had slept in his clothes for three nights, he had a swollen left hand and arm which he was reluctant to show. In the local casualty department he was found to have a left Colles' fracture and a fractured left olecranon, he was raw with sweating in the axilla and his shirt and jumper had to be cut from him. The physiotherapist was contacted by the orthopaedic department and asked to manage the arm adjusting the splint and bandaging as necessary to accommodate the gross swelling and advising the patient and nursing staff on general care.

Some old clothing was found which could be cut to allow Mr. *N* to wear the back slab and sling outside his clothes. This was important to remind his more vigorous companions on the ward that he must not be knocked and also to encourage Mr. *N* to move. Mr. *N* came of his own accord to the physiotherapy department each morning and a blind eye was turned to his erratic time keeping. He was always welcomed positively whatever the time and he responded well. Mr. *N* worked hard to reduce the swelling in his fingers with his arm in elevation on pillows and allowed the physiotherapist to support his arm while he moved his shoulder.

Mr. *N*'s initial appearance, drooling with tardive dyskinesia and slurred speech, coughing on a cigarette, with ash, spittle and breakfast trailing down his stubbly chin made him an unattractive prospect for the physiotherapist. However, underneath his reserve was a gentle uncomplaining conscientious man who increasingly related and responded to advice. Long after Mr. *N* was better he still took the initiative in greeting the physiotherapist by her first name when he passed her in the hospital corridor, though he appeared not to notice others whom he must have known well. The physiotherapist was gratified to feel that not only had she helped to heal his arm but that he related positively to her in his subsequent everyday life rather than withdrawing into himself again.

Epilepsy

Epilepsy is caused by an abnormal electrical discharge in the brain. The sufferer experiences repeated fits (or convulsions) of varying length and severity. The majority of epileptics are able to live normally in the community aided by drug therapy. A small proportion of people with epilepsy deteriorate mentally and physically and are sometimes admitted to a psychiatric hospital. The epileptic patient may be subject to minor episodes, '*petit mal*' attacks, where he seems briefly to lose concentration, perhaps dropping what he is holding, or losing the thread of a conversation. These attacks only last for a few seconds and occur only in the young. Major fits or *'grand mal'* seizures, may result in a total loss of consciousness, falling to the ground and stiffness followed by violent twitching and cyanosis. The patient may foam at the mouth and is often incontinent. Subsequently the patient may sleep deeply sometimes for many hours and may be amnesic and disorientated.

The violence of a fall during a seizure results in head and other injuries and the subsequent deep sleep can initiate a chest infection in a patient who has inhaled saliva or food during a fit. Repeated, severe, and frequent fits can lead to a gradual impairment of mobility and brain damage.

Case History (4.6)

Mr. O had lived as a young man in a colony for epileptics which he had enjoyed. The colony had been disbanded and having no known relatives Mr. O had been placed in a psychiatric hospital. He was now 55 years old and on a heavy dependency ward. Mr. O's fits were so violent that he had sustained many severe injuries over the years. It was necessary for him to use a wheelchair as his balance had become too poor for him to stand unsupported even with a walking aid. Mr. O joined in a movement group from his chair and was stood up between two people as often as possible. The physiotherapist was frequently needed to help clear Mr. O's chest because chest infections often followed severe fits and long sleeps. Mr. O was brave and cheerful and even when too ill to speak coherently, signed to his carers with a smile and thumbs-up sign.

Huntington's Chorea

Huntington's chorea is a hereditary disease resulting in degenerative changes in the frontal areas of the brain and the corpus striatum. The disease usually manifests itself in early middle age when the patient has already produced a family. It is more common in the more remote areas of the country such as East Anglia and the Fens in England, where intermarriage in small communities is more likely.

Jerky, athetochoreiform movements of the upper limbs

and face are characteristic and the sufferer becomes increasingly emotionally unstable and irritable. As the disease progresses the whole body is gradually affected. Speech, gait and behaviour deteriorate until the patient is demented, mute and has a twitching body. Fifty per cent of the children of sufferers are likely to have inherited the condition and if they marry and have children at a young age then the original carrier may have had grandchildren before the disease manifests itself in the grandparent. Careful genetic counselling is essential for the families of sufferers who often need considerable emotional support. The illness carries a high risk of suicide.

There is little written help available to physiotherapists involved in helping patients with Huntington's chorea with their gross physical problems.

There is a self help association for sufferers and their families in the United Kingdom called COMBAT.[2] One centre specifically for the treatment of Huntington's chorea is the Arthur Preston Care Centre in Australia.[3] Here the physiotherapists have been able to devise a treatment scheme suitable for all stages of the illness. The Australian scheme includes imaginative group movement work which helps to maintain physical ability and combat the inevitable weakness and the perceptual defects experienced. It also includes chest physiotherapy, in particular postural drainage to help eliminate secretions. The disease which affects the upper limbs and facial muscles initially, causes difficulties in coughing and swallowing. A patient can easily choke and inhale food or be unable to cough up phlegm unless aided.

Case History (4.7)

Mr. *P* was 67 and lived at home with his wife. He attended a day centre three times a week. Mr. *P* walked with an erratic wandering gait, his shoulders and arms writhed as he moved and his head twisted to one side, he liked to be able to hold the hand of his companion as he walked. Mr. *P* was prone to chest infections and had chronic bronchitis. His cheeks were hollowed and he made constant chewing movements and dribbled. Mr. *P* often arrived at the day centre in some distress because of blocked airways. He was sometimes aggressive with his wife and unwilling to let her help him with any form of postural drainage. She was herself elderly and frail. A short tip on a tilt table with accompanying chest vibrations always cleared Mr. P's chest quickly and gave him considerable relief.

Teaching relaxation can help reduce involuntary movements and facial relaxation. Massage and mouth closing exercises may help patients with dribbling and swallowing problems.

An active programme of rehabilitation therapy based on Bobath techniques can be attempted with a limited number of highly motivated patients, but in view of the degenerative nature of the disease and the mental changes induced success is likely to be limited.

Late Stage and Progressive Neurological Conditions

Decreasing independence and mobility sometimes combined with increasingly erratic behaviour are a problem to treat positively. The following case history illustrates the difficulty faced by large institutions in providing suitable facilities for the care of rarer diseases.

Case History (4.8)

Mr. Q was a 66-year-old man suffering from Huntington's chorea. He lived on an active heavy dependency ward which was upstairs. Mr. Q's behaviour was unpredictable but on the whole he was aggressively independent. He got around in bursts of movement often coming to a stop by banging into a wall or falling over a chair. In the hospital corridors he made abrupt turns at inappropriate places and more than once was so winded by a fall that he was taken back to his ward in a wheelchair.

Mr. Q began to have difficulty in feeding himself. His spoon missed his mouth and what little food reached his mouth he had difficulty swallowing. He violently resisted all assistance. Eventually emaciated and unable to walk he was admitted to the hospital sick bay for the treatment of sores on his knees where they rubbed together continually as he crossed his legs. In the sick bay Mr. Q was more cooperative. He allowed nurses to help him feed and the physiotherapists were able to mobilise him as he gained strength.

On return to his ward Mr. Q took to crashing around again. In particular he would throw himself out of bed at night and hurl himself down the stairs. An urgent request was made for Mr. Q to be transferred to a ground floor ward for his own safety. In this particular hospital all the downstairs wards were geriatric wards with far less active programmes than the ward he was leaving. Mr. Q however was old enough to be accepted on a geriatric ward and he went to one which housed many disturbed old people in their eighties with late stage senile dementia.

Mr. Q became severely depressed and miserable, withdrawn and unwilling to join in activities. His speech was rarely intelligible and he was unable to relate to other patients on the ward. The move had emphasised his deterioration. Mr. Q regularly refused to join in the music and movement session run by the physiotherapist on the ward although just occasionally he would accept an invitation to dance and enjoy a familiar waltz around the floor.

Seating and Sleeping of Huntington's Chorea Patients

The seating of Huntington's chorea patients in late stages of the disease is very difficult. The patients wriggle and writhe and eventually slide onto the floor. Ordinary chairs are too upright, restraints rub and chafe, sag bags, hammocks and bucket seat chairs promote flexion deformities. In addition safe beds have also to be provided and the violent writhing of a patient can result in bruising if conventional cot sides are used.

Case History (4.9)

Mrs. R was only 45 but she was living on a small geriatric ward as there were no facilities for younger patients in her extreme state. Mrs. R was mute and depressed. She could walk between two nurses and enjoyed doing so. Mrs. R loathed group work and if asked to join in a group, would sit and weep copiously. Mrs. R loved to be taken out of the ward into the gardens but she liked a weekly coach trip in the surrounding countryside best of all. Eventually Mrs. R's writhing movements meant that she could no longer sit safely in a coach seat or even an ordinary wheelchair. She was well aware which morning was coach trip morning and started to scream and cry from breakfast time onwards for fear she could not go.

The physiotherapist took Mrs *R* on a stretcher to the local wheelchair clinic. Here she was fitted with the largest size of wheelchair designed for cerebral palsied children. Padded headrest and padded footbox were necessary. As the chair could be reclined back Mrs. *R* no longer slipped out when being pushed. This wheelchair could also be taken on the hospital's coach. Subsequently Mrs. *R* was managed in a combination of bucket arm chair and wheelchair. When weather permitted she lay prone on a mattress in the garden. Sleeping was also a problem and the hospital carpenter and the upholsterer designed and made a padded head board and sides which fitted round a mattress on the floor, a system subsequently used for two other similar patients.

Head Injuries

Scattered throughout the psychiatric hospitals are a number of young patients who have severe brain damage due to head injuries. These are the patients whose subsequent behavioural disabilities cause them to be rejected by other caring institutions. They usually have gross residual physical disability also. Some patients are successfully managed in units specialising in the care of head injuries. The physiotherapist may also be involved in units which practice a token economy system for acceptable behaviour. In this system a patient earns tokens for simple tasks such as combing hair each morning. These tokens can then be exchanged by the patient for meals, cigarettes or other rewards. Token economy wards need a very high staff patient ratio to work properly and the patients need much attention and encouragement. It follows that such a system is expensive to run and hospital finances may not allow for this. In effect the majority of severely disturbed patients with head injuries are managed on heavy dependency wards and the nursing staff bear the brunt of any antisocial behaviour and patiently work to provide simple purposeful routines to aid maximum independence. These patients may have received a great deal of physical treatment before their placement, however patients with head injuries often go on improving for a very long time and the physiotherapist continues to have an important role in the maintenance of existing ability and the continued improvement of the head injured patient.

If a patient is not receiving specific physiotherapy, the physiotherapist should monitor the patient's physical ability through ward movement groups and regular visits to the ward. Should a problem arise the physiotherapist who is already known to the patient will find it easier to build up a relationship of trust and understanding if specific treatment becomes necessary. Severely handicapped patients quickly regress physically without constant encouragement.

Case History (4.10)

Mr. S had suffered brain damage due to anoxia following an attempt to hang himself when he was in his late teens. He was now 27 and living on a heavy dependency ward. Mr. S could not speak but uttered blood-curdling screams if aroused. He was ataxic and would only walk independently pushing his wheelchair which he sometimes shoved violently across the ward. He was young, powerful and frustrated. His only real pleasure was in feeding himself which he could manage with adapted utensils. He did this noisily and messily. Mr. S had had a great deal of physical rehabilitation before his admission to a psychiatric unit. The nursing staff managed him on a simple routine to which he was well adjusted. Suddenly one day Mr. S started to refuse to walk with his wheelchair. He stood legs apart screaming and throwing his arms apart but would not budge. After a week the nursing staff were desparate and the charge nurse approached the physiotherapist to see if she could help.

It was agreed that Mr. S would be brought in his wheelchair to the physiotherapy department by a nurse whom he knew and trusted. The nurse would stay during the session as Mr. S did not know the physiotherapist. As soon as Mr. S came into the department he started screaming, obviously frustrated. His chair was wheeled to the parallel bars and Mr. S grabbed them and walked down and back. Mr. S remembered what a physiotherapy department was. This still did not solve the problem as he would walk in the department but not on the ward.

The department was quiet and peaceful and the ward full of bustle. The physiotherapist wondered if this was the problem and decided to try walking with Mr. S back to his ward. Mr. S would hold the hand rail running along the corridor wall, the physiotherapist would support his other side and the nurse followed reassuringly behind with the wheelchair. Initially it was quiet and all went well but a group of patients started to approach noisily. Mr. S went rigid and one look at his face, a picture of terror, told the story. Mr. S was afraid to walk where there were others.

The physiotherapist supported Mr. S protectively and gently talked to him to reassure him, he calmed down and walked on when the people had passed. Each time people approached from behind or in front Mr. S was stopped and soothingly reassured. After about a fortnight Mr. S started to be able to practise pushing his chair on the ward again and all was back to normal. It was decided that another patient had frightened Mrs. S by pushing him, or by being aggressive in some way and his fear of falling which was always evident had frightened him into immobility.

Mental Impairment

A proportion of patients being cared for by the psychiatric services are bordering on mental impairment (mental handicap). These people are not so handicapped that they cannot cope with independent life but, as with children, if small things go wrong they are reduced to an extreme state of anxiety and inability to cope.

While such people should be managed in the community many were originally placed in the old-style mental institutions. Work is progressing to teach these old people to live independently again. Any incidental physical therapy these patients need must be very simple and basic. Anxiety and panic need a calm approach and a short relaxation session may be necessary as a preliminary to treatment. Such patients' aches and pains may be a physical expression of their mental illness so careful assessment is needed.

Other Conditions

The physiotherapist must be versatile enough to meet the needs of a very wide variety of conditions. Of the many neurological illnesses which may be encountered neurosyphilis still occurs. The high stepping gait of a patient with tabes dorsalis walking past in the corridor should instantly alert the physiotherapist to the problems of lack of sensation, ill-fitting shoes and subsequent sores which will not heal.

A patient may have suffered an amputation or paraplegia and specialist advice on management will be expected from the physiotherapy department.

Above all the physiotherapist working with the chronically mentally ill must be a good versatile experienced generalist with plenty of initiative to give a strong lead to others on the physical side of caring.

References

1. Clark D. H. (1981). *Social Therapy in Psychiatry* (pp. 45–64). London: Churchill Livingstone.
2. *The Association to Combat Huntington's Chorea* Theydon Road, Epping, Essex, CM16 4DX. England.
3. *Arthur Preston Care Centre for Huntington's Disease* Marys Mount, 27 Yarrbat Avenue, Balwyn 3103, Melbourne, Australia.

Further Reading

Barton R. (1966). *Institutional Neurosis*. Bristol: John Wright.

Jones M. (1953). *The Therapeutic Community*. New York: N.Y. Basic Books.

Caplow Linder E., Harpaz L., Samberg S. (1979). Expressive activities for older adults. In *Therapeutic Dance/Movement*. London: Human Science Press.

Evans C. D. (1981). *Rehabilitation After Severe Head Injury*. London: Churchill Livingstone.

Wilson M. (1983). *Occupational Therapy in Long Term Psychiatry*. London: Churchill Livingstone.

Benson D. F., Blumer D. (1975). *Psychiatric Aspects of Neurological Disease*. Orlando, California: Grune and Stratton.

5

Mental Illness in the Elderly

It is clearly stated in the important document on developing services for the mentally ill elderly, 'The Rising Tide'[1], that the specialist physiotherapist should be a key member of a team working with the mentally ill elderly. Nevertheless, the physiotherapy profession as a whole is reluctant to venture into this role. Those who do, find the scope for their talents very satisfying. Not only does the individual physiotherapist with initiative have the opportunity to develop new areas of interest in her role as a member of this team, but for those with enquiring minds the opportunities for research projects are many. Psychogeriatrics has a low priority in the syllabus in the schools of physiotherapy, despite the fact that one-quarter of all patients admitted to psychiatric wards are over 65 years old and all these people suffer from the same physical problems of ageing as those in general and geriatric units.

Care of the old and infirm is a major growth area for the developed world. Currently about 14% of the population in the United Kingdom is aged over 65[2]. This proportion is increasing as the birth rate declines and as modern social conditions and medical knowledge enable more people to live into old age.

Those unfamiliar with the psychiatric problems of the old may hold a false impression that senile dementia is the only major problem for the consultant psychogeriatrician. This is not so. Long-term care of the severely demented is important, and a survey in 1964[3] revealed that 10% of those aged over 65 suffer some degree of dementia, however 15% of those surveyed suffered from some form of neurotic illness, such as depression or anxiety. The statistics for suicide will reveal that those over 65 account for one-third of the annual suicides in the United Kingdom.[4]

Provision of care for the mentally ill elderly varies from region to region. Current trends and recommendations in health care place the bulk of the work firmly in the community, backed up by day centres.[1] The more acutely ill are provided for in specialist psychogeriatric units at hospitals where patients may be assessed and receive medical treatments. In principle, ward units for those with dementia are separate from those with other mental illnesses. It is cruel to admit a patient with depression to a ward full of people suffering from dementia and the vision of those with such disordered behaviour can only serve to depress the patient further.

The psychogeriatric unit may also provide beds for a holiday relief scheme, chronic long-term care beds and possibly a terminal care unit.

Psychiatric Disorders in the Elderly

There are two major areas of mental disorder in the elderly, those whose illness is of organic origin and those with psychiatric illness. A third minor category includes those with personality disorders which develop in old age.

Organic Diseases

Organic disease is more often the cause of mental illness in the elderly than in the young, due to processes of ageing and physical deterioration.

Dementia

The two major forms of dementia which affect the elderly are Alzheimer-type disease and multi-infarct dementia. To date drugs, developed specifically to combat the progressive degeneration of the brain in dementia are largely unsuccessful.[5] Present methods of treatment are founded on the concept of maintaining independence and a reasonable quality of life for the patient within the community, together with practical support for caring relatives. Reality orientation is generally practised with dementing patients (*see* Chapter 9).

Alzheimer-type Disease (Senile Dementia)

Alzheimer-type disease, sometimes known as senile dementia, is caused by the increasing development of senile plaques in the ageing brain. Forgetfulness is usually the earliest sign of senile dementia. The insidious nature of the onset of the illness and the acceptance by the general public that older people become less reliable in their habits as a matter of course, may mean that a family does not realise that their elderly relative has early dementia. It is when behaviour becomes illogical or outbursts of aggression or incontinence make life intolerable for others that help may be sought by the carers. Those living alone may become reclusive, or wander in the streets at inappropriate times until an accident or anxious neighbours alert the authorities.

The slow destruction of brain tissue in this disease does not produce gross motor or neurological problems in the early stages. The patient remains physically able but has an inability to recognise everyday objects and situations. The elderly person continually getting up from the chair and wandering around unable to sit down again because they do not recognise what a chair is, is a common phenomenon.

Physiotherapy in Alzheimer-type Disease

The physiotherapist is most likely to be asked to assess a patient with early Alzheimer-type disease in order to help the team define which functional disabilities are due to loss of cognitive brain power and which due to other specific physical causes. During later stages of the illness the physiotherapist may be increasingly involved in helping to solve such problems and advising relatives and nurses on appropriate care.

Case History (5.1)

Mrs. *T* was an 82-year-old widow. She had been admitted to an assessment ward from a local authority home because of her bouts of aggressive behaviour and because she was having repeated falls. Mrs. *T* was indeed aggressive if approached suddenly but if approached gently with soothing talk she was quiet and seemed attentive. She was unable to talk coherently.

The physiotherapist was asked to assess Mrs. *T*'s mobility. She could walk well and had reasonably strong arms and legs, but her steps were hesitant and after standing for some time in one place she would often just collapse in a heap. Mrs *T* was much more confident on the arm of the physiotherapist. However, in front of a chair she was completely unable to coordinate turning and sitting. Simple visual tests revealed that Mrs. *T* had peripheral vision only but even if a chair was placed in Mrs. *T*'s line of vision she did not relate to it but stood or tottered on until she tripped or fell. Experiments using a walking aid were equally useless as she just let go of the aid, wandered forwards and fell over it.

It became obvious that a combination of visual impairment and a lack of ability to recognise everyday objects was the basic cause of falling. The physiotherapist recommended to the ward team that in order for Mrs. *T* to stay mobile safely she needed constant monitoring when walking. This was not possible in her previous accommodation and she was found a place on a long-stay psychogeriatric ward with a high ratio of nurses to patients. In this way it was possible to monitor her aimless walking and for someone to be more readily on hand if she seemed close to collapse. Mrs. *T*'s aggressive outbursts diminished in the atmosphere of closer care probably because she felt more secure in her environment.

Case History (5.2)

Mrs. *U* aged 79 had suffered from senile dementia for several years. She was an aimless wanderer but could feed herself and sit down safely. She was unable to speak coherently. The long-term psychogeriatric ward which was her home, had a positive approach to keeping patients mobile. Mrs. *U* became ill with a severe cold and was confined to bed for a few days. When she was well enough to get up she did not recover her ability to walk. Normally the nursing staff would expect to assist a patient to walk after a short stay in bed but Mrs. *U*'s ability did not improve. The charge nurse asked the physiotherapist's advice.

Mrs. U had a habit of rubbing parts of the body with her hands as she sat or walked. It was noticed that the rubbing had concentrated itself on the knees. The physiotherapist examined Mrs. U and was pushed off when she tried to examine her knees. Mrs. U was obviously unable to straighten her knees completely and although they were not noticably warm to touch it seemed they were the focus of some pain. The psychiatrist agreed to prescribe a mild pain killer and the physiotherapist decided to give Mrs. U regular treatment.

Mrs. U was brought to the physiotherapy department and sat on a wide couch. She was rather agitated but biddable. It was not possible to test Mrs. U's skin sensation so no specific heat or cold treatment could be given. The physiotherapist switched on a large heat lamp and let it play on herself and Mrs. U together as she sat on the couch with her. Mrs. U liked this, she smiled and stopped her ceaseless rubbing, stretching her arm towards the lamp.

Warm and comfortable Mrs. U allowed the physiotherapist to rhythmically bend and stretch her knees gently. She relaxed and began to join in the movement. Eventually Mrs. U was able to straighten her knees on the bed.

The lamp was switched off and Mrs. U was stood up between two people. She took a few steps leaning on them heavily. The physiotherapist talked to the nurses giving them advice on positioning and helping Mrs. U move. Mrs. U was unable to grasp the function of a walking aid but soon became willing to walk leaning on two people. The physiotherapy was continued for two weeks until Mrs. U no longer held her knees flexed on the couch, and she stopped the incessant rubbing of her knees. It took four weeks for Mrs. U to walk independently again.

Multi-infarct Dementia (Cerebrovascular Dementia)

Multi-infarct dementia is caused by arteriosclerosis in the cerebral blood vessels. It is the second major form of dementia, characterised by the sudden production of major neurological problems such as blackouts, convulsions or paralysis. A patient may recover from an incident quickly when a cerebral artery is blocked by a clot which later moves on or is absorbed. On the other hand the blockage may persist causing permanent brain damage.

Such patients offer a confusing pattern of symptoms to the physiotherapist used to the more regular pattern of a stroke. One arm or leg may be spastic for a few days then recover suddenly and the strength of muscular spasm may vary considerably from day to day.

Physiotherapy for Multi-infarct Dementia

The physiotherapist has a very important role in the care of these patients. They are particularly prone to contracture and the importance of maintaining full ranges of movement during spastic episodes is emphasised if a patient recovers, but is left with a contracture. Two other points have to be considered, first that particularly if a patient is experiencing fits frequently it is virtually impossible to prevent some degree of contracture. Conscientious nursing and physiotherapy staff may worry about their failure in this respect but some of the spasms are exceptionally strong. Second, because pain accompanies spasm then the patient who cannot speak may hit out, scratch or attempt to bite someone who seems to be causing that pain. Soothing talk, stroking, a comforting arm and very gentle progression are all important. Handling is a very important part of caring for those who live in confusion and cannot communicate. The physiotherapist, skilled in the art of how to support injured and painful limbs will find that patients soon sense this and become calmer and more cooperative.

Case History (5.3)

Mrs. *V* was only 62 and was cared for by her husband at home. She had been suffering from multi-infarct dementia for two years. Mrs. *V* had always been a very active and self sufficient woman, who had supervised the running of a large office.

Her husband was very caring but had difficulty in adjusting to her total dependence and readily panicked when faced with problems over his wife.

Mrs. *V* had a series of 'stroke' type incidents and blackouts from which she recovered. At home she became less and less mobile. The more agitated her husband became over this, the worse Mrs. *V* became. Her speech was garbled but she often swore clearly at her husband.

The psychogeriatrician visited the couple and decided to admit Mrs. *V* to help to break the cycle of immobility and anxiety, and to see if Mrs. *V* and her husband would benefit from a holiday relief scheme. As part of the team the physiotherapist arranged to assess Mrs. *V* physically and talk to her husband about any mobility problems she was having at home.

At the time Mrs. *V* had a mild spastic diplegia, her arms appeared to be normal and she tried hard to concentrate on the physiotherapy. She was rigid and wary when standing and was wearing a pair of very high heeled shoes. Mrs. *V*'s gait was hesitant and changes in floor colouring confused her, she would try and step high over a dark patch as if it were a step. Mrs. *V* could recognise a chair but in common with many in her condition, she would forget to turn round in front of the chair before sitting down. Mrs. *V*'s ability diminished markedly in the presence of her husband. As she tried to do things he fidgeted round her getting increasingly agitated. Mrs. *V* responded by becoming rooted to the spot, jerkily pushing him off, her normally garbled speech crystallising into a swear word.

The physiotherapist and the rest of the ward team spent some time with Mrs. *V*'s husband helping him to see what he was doing and encouraging him to become calmer. The physiotherapist showed him how she was able to walk with Mrs *V* and climb stairs, sit down and negotiate the toilet. Mrs. *V*'s husband watched from a distance and refrained from commenting, noticing how the calm atmosphere helped. He was then shown how to hold Mrs. *V* confidently and where to stand to give reassurance especially on the stairs. He learned not to hurry Mrs. *V* and gradually their relationship improved. A local shoe shop allowed Mrs. *V*'s husband to bring in a selection of shoes and the physiotherapist helped to choose a suitable pair.

It was decided to admit Mrs. *V* to the relief scheme and she would stay on the relief ward for one week in every six to give her husband a break at home. This worked well and Mrs. *V*'s husband discussed any ongoing problems each time she was admitted. During that week of admission the physiotherapist reviewed Mrs. *V*'s mobility and helped with advice to the husband. The physiotherapist did not have a brief to do home visits but the department telephone number was given to Mrs. *V*'s husband in case of problems. He rarely used this and when he did his problem was usually of his own making due to impatience or agitation. A few words of friendly advice from a professional who knew the situation was all that was needed and the husband felt able to cope again.

Toxic Confusional States

A toxic confusional state may be also referred to as an acute organic psychosis or as delirium. This condition is common in the frail elderly and results in the patient becoming rapidly disorientated. The patient in a confused state is just as likely to be met in a general hospital ward as in a psychiatric unit. The most common cause of the condition is an adverse reaction to drugs, but other causes include anoxia, acute infection, metabolic disorder, endocrine disorder, diseases of the central nervous system, vitamin deficiency and alcohol withdrawal. The physiotherapist will be most familiar with the patient who becomes acutely confused due to anoxia as a result of respiratory disease.

Physiotherapy

The maintenance of mobility, the prevention of contractures and pressure sores, and the clearing of airways are the important factors for the physiotherapist to bear in mind. Patients often recover within a few days and the prevention of additional problems such as chest infections can be aided by regular physiotherapy.

Neurological Illnesses

The late stages of many progressive neurological disorders may be encountered in psychogeriatric units, as resulting brain damage produces disordered or antisocial behaviour. The physiotherapist must expect to meet some of the more rare conditions such as Huntington's chorea (*see* Chapter 4) and neurosyphilis. More commonly those with parkinson's disease, late stage multiple sclerosis or head injury are encountered.

Physiotherapy

The physiotherapist will be familiar with the main problems of the major neurological disorders. The treatments offered need to be adjusted to enable the patient to live a purposeful life within the bounds of disability. Maintenance of physical ability for as long as possible within the limits of the disease is the major goal. The prevention of pain due to contractures is important. Many patients may be severely depressed by their condition and resist help, feeling it to be pointless. Combined, consistent care routines on the part of the whole ward team help to support the patient in his desperation. Remembering that many unqualified nursing helpers provide basic care on long-term wards, the physiotherapist will frequently and patiently need to explain the importance of positioning, and maintaining mobility.

Selected Depressive Disorders

Depression

Depression is a major psychiatric illness of old age. Depression in the elderly is often more entrenched than in younger persons and therefore more difficult to treat successfully. Coming to terms with the ageing process, loss of job, reduced status, bereavement and illness are typical of the environmental factors contributing to a bout of depression. The depressed elderly attach little value to their own worth in society and are prey to a variety of hypochondriacal symptoms. Those whose depression is severe may have delusions of persecution, guilt or ill health and express considerable hostility to those trying to help.

One-third of successful suicide attempts are in the over 65 age group with men predominating. Attempted suicide is less common than in younger age groups. The majority of elderly people with mild depression are treated with antidepressive drugs by their general practitioners. Only those with more severe problems are referred to the psychogeriatrician. Therefore the physiotherapist attached to a psychogeriatric unit is more likely to encounter those patients with the worst intractable depressions.

Manic Depressive Psychosis

A small number of patients suffer from manic depression. Their treatment is the same as for younger patients.

Depressive Pseudodementia

Some patients who are severely depressed may present with the symptoms of senile dementia. This is a major diagnostic problem for the psychiatrist, who will be concerned to avoid placing a depressive patient with patients who are dementing. In addition depression is often a factor in the early stages of senile dementia which further complicates the issue. Careful psychological tests can usually resolve the problem promptly.

Treatment of depression in the elderly is by drug therapy or ECT with supportive group or psychotherapy. Even where treatment is initially successful there is a high relapse rate for depressive illness in the elderly.

Physiotherapy for the Depressed Elderly

Physical Problems

Physical illness is often one of the underlying causes of depression in the elderly. However, the physiotherapist needs to be alert to the possibilities of the concealed physical disability. This is particularly common in the case of the recent widow who finds herself doing heavy chores formerly performed by the husband such as carrying in the coal for the fire, or as in the following case history, a much lighter job.

Case History (5.4)

A 75-year-old widow, Mrs. *W* with rheumatoid arthritis had lived alone for three months since the death of her husband. She used a walking frame in her bungalow and attended a geriatric day centre. To all intents and purposes Mrs. *W* seemed to be coping well with her problems. She was quiet, obliging and undemanding at the centre. One morning Mrs. *W* was found unconscious by her home help, she had taken an overdose of the tablets prescribed for her arthritis. Mrs. *W* was admitted to an acute psychiatric ward where it transpired that she had struggled hard to cope with her bereavement, presenting a picture of being able to manage, but the last straw had been the inability to lift a hot teapot or kettle to make a cup of tea. Mrs. *W*'s husband had always done this. One evening she had dropped the teapot and in desperation took an overdose of pills. The physiotherapist and the occupational therapist worked together with Mrs. *W* and between them they helped her to solve her immediate physical problems. Both professionals were alerted to the need to be especially attentive to the seemingly minor needs of the recently bereaved.

Debility

The severely depressed elderly neglect themselves and become debilitated as a result of inadequate diet. Subsequently they may become immobile and suffer from chest infections. The importance of regular exercise cannot be stressed enough. However, a very gentle approach is needed and an over hearty physiotherapist will not form a good relationship with her patient.

Case History (5.5)

Mrs. *X* was 72 and widowed. She lived in a local authority home. Mrs. *X* had had a stroke four years previously resulting in a mild left hemiplegia. She was able to walk unaided and cope with the basic essentials of daily life and was not mentally impaired. Mrs. *X* became increasingly depressed, she refused to walk, eat or help herself. She began to lose weight at the home. She was aggressive with staff and other residents and insisted she saw no point in their caring.

Mrs. *X* was admitted to an acute psychogeriatric assessment ward with a psychotic depression. Her immobility required the immediate attention of the physiotherapist who was aggressively rebuffed with such phrases as 'What's the point?' and 'I tell you it's not worth it'. Mrs. X accused her carers of wanting to make life more of a misery.

The physiotherapist discovered an indirect approach to treatment worked best, treating others on the ward first and then perhaps quietly sitting beside Mrs. X. Mrs. X was then expected to make the first approach 'I suppose you want me to come with you? Well, there's no point'. After carrying on in this vein for some while Mrs. X would usually say 'Well, I can't see the point, but you might as well get on with it'. The physiotherapist would then be allowed to stretch the stiff arm and leg and begin to assist Mrs. X towards walking independently.

The nursing and occupational therapy staff had to be similarly patient over mealtimes and dressing practice. Gradually Mrs. X became mobile again but remained aggressively depressed despite drug therapy. Subsequently the physiotherapy helper kept a regular watch on Mrs. X's mobility and was brusquely tolerated by Mrs. X.

Chest Infection

Chest infections are a frequent complication of depressive illness in the elderly. They can contribute to confusional states and prevent prompt treatment by ECT if indicated. The physiotherapist will be asked to assess and treat those whom she feels she can benefit.

Neurosis

Anxiety states, phobias, obsessive states and hyperventilation attacks are some of the more common manifestations of neurosis in the elderly. Such states usually coexist with depressive illness. Some patients who have had a long history of neurosis throughout life have learned to live through their problems. Others present with new symptoms having previously had no history of neurosis.

Physiotherapy

The physiotherapist will need to assess and treat those

whose extreme anxiety causes them to hyperventilate and panic if required to walk independently. Every physiotherapist is familiar with the patient who works herself into a state of agitation a few steps from the chair and sits on the floor. Such patients are extremely accident prone and if they happen to fall and fracture a hip in the process, this only serves to reinforce the panic. Breaking the cycle of agitation and panic on attempts to mobilise require great fortitude and patience on the part of the physiotherapist and all staff who are involved.

Case History (5.6)

Mrs. Y aged 78 was mildly depressed and had been cared for in her daughter's house for many years. Mrs. Y became increasingly agitated and refused to get up and move around the house even with a stick or walking aid. After taking a few steps she would start to hyperventilate, crying, and saying that she could not go on. She would then collapse in a heap on the floor saying that she was too old.

Mrs. Y's daughter could not cope and Mrs. Y was admitted for assessment and treatment. Mrs. Y began drug therapy and became calmer. The physiotherapist started to mobilise her in a quiet department. Mrs. Y refused to take any weight through her knees and so was stood in gentle stages using a tilt table. Gradually she began to take a few steps without panic using a walking aid. In the bustle of the ward Mrs Y still refused to stand without panicking. The nursing staff took turns in coming to the physiotherapy department, and helped her walk using the parallel bars and her frame.

Quiet times were chosen to encourage Mrs. Y to walk on the ward and gradually she began to make short trips, vocally calmed by whoever was accompanying her. Typically Mrs. Y was more likely to have a panic attack if more than one professional was giving her attention. The less help given the more likely Mrs. Y was to achieve her goal though often with a great display of agitation.

One day Mrs. Y did slip and fall, fracturing the right neck of her femur. She had a Thompson's prosthesis inserted and the physiotherapist started again. Mrs. Y was eventually transferred to a long-stay ward where the patients were active and mobile. She remained depressed and agitated, able to walk with a walking frame, at risk of falling if left alone and prone to dramatic displays if helped.

Paranoid States

Paranoid states commonly feature in parallel with other illnesses in the elderly. Deafness and failure of vision exacerbate the problem and patients may be acutely suspicious of all they hear or see especially in unfamiliar surroundings. A patient may believe he is being persecuted or robbed by nurses or other patients. These feelings can easily induce aggressive behaviour of which the physiotherapist must be aware. The physiotherapist should not let herself be drawn into arguments with the patient about the rights and wrongs of these paranoid delusions but try and maintain a sympathetic neutrality.

Personality Disorders

Some old people, often without mental illness become eccentric, dirty uncommunicative and stubborn. It is difficult to consider these people as ill. They are unlikely to change their ways and are often uncomfortable companions and neighbours. Pleas for help for the old person are in reality pleas from the relatives or neighbours for their release from the burden of the antisocial behaviour. A number of elderly people in this condition are admitted to psychogeriatric wards because these are the only places where the old person will be tolerated.

A Comprehensive Physiotherapy Service for the Mentally Ill Elderly

A comprehensive physiotherapy service for the mentally ill elderly should be an integral part of the whole service, complementing other members of the psychogeriatric team. The physiotherapist needs easy access to patients, whether in hospital or the community, to all members of the team and to the relatives of patients. Where community and hospital budgets are held seperately, units will need to be specially vigilant that demarcation does not impair the continuity of care for the patient.

The psychogeriatric team will be led by a consultant psychogeriatrician backed by a team specialising in different aspects of care. The psychiatric nurse is the main stay of this service with back up from social workers, psychologists, occupational therapists and physiotherapists. Other professions such as chiropody and dietetics will also play a prominent role.

Patterns of psychogeriatric care are still evolving but at the present time the core of the unit will probably be the psychogeriatric assessment ward. By no means all or even the majority of patients will pass through this unit but it is a meeting of the ways for staff involved in hospital and community care. While the assessment unit influences the placing of patients and their treatment, the day centre is often the common bond for patients whether living at home or in care.

The Role of the Physiotherapist

Ideally a superintendent or senior physiotherapist in charge of a psychogeriatric unit should have overall control of the physiotherapy services to that specialty in the hospital, day centre and in the community in order to coordinate services efficiently. In practice community physiotherapy services in some areas are still minimal and may be funded separately. The problem of who should do home visits and assessments has to be solved according to local conditions.

Practical advice on physical problems is much appreciated by both medical and nursing staff on the psychogeriatric team. It must always be noted that some psychiatric nurses do not do a general nurse training therefore they need more help and guidance over the management of physical problems. In addition, a high proportion of nursing helpers are used in psychogeriatric wards and local authority homes. Their knowledge of the body and its functions is very limited and an understanding of basic facts such as the names of bones or the normal range of movement of a joint cannot be assumed. The physiotherapist must remember this when teaching or leaving instructions.

The approach of the physiotherapist working in a psychogeriatric unit needs to be sympathetic especially with those who are depressed. Much talking and touching goes on in such a unit. Patients and staff will not discriminate between those whose role is mainly to talk and those who do a job and expect to move on. The physiotherapist will be expected to take time, to listen, to comfort and give mental as well as physical support as a routine part of the work. The basic physiotherapy remains the same. The skill is in adapting to the extremes of mental stress and finding a way to work through and achieve a positive outcome.

Physiotherapy on a Psychogeriatric Assessment Ward

Patients admitted to a psychogeriatric assessment ward may be well known to community staff or they may have been visited at home by the consultant. The assessment ward should be visited by a physiotherapist every day in order to tackle a new patient's problems as soon as is practicable.

The patients admitted to this ward will probably be experiencing an acute mental crisis. Many will be severely depressed. Ideally there will be separate assessment units for those with the problems of senile dementia but this is not always possible. Patients on the assessment ward may be acutely confused by their change of environment and present negative attitudes which express their fear, hostility or resentment on admission. The ward needs to have a calm, orderly and friendly atmosphere. Extra tolerance and understanding is required for the patient who finds it is four times as far to the toilet as at home and does not make it in time. Every effort will have been made to minimise this type of inconvenience but the many old buildings in use make provision of more homely facilities difficult. The main areas of work for the physiotherapist are discussed below.

Physical Assessment

A clear indication of the physical abilities and potential of a patient is required for future planning. A hospital may use formal assessment forms but precise physical assessment can be very difficult with an unresponding or hostile patient. Complicated assessment forms can be patiently filled in and then filed away in the notes unread by other staff. One way to avoid this is to write a brief statement on physical ability in the doctor's notes where it will be read and to attend ward rounds regularly.

The physiotherapist can then keep more detailed records in the department for future comparisons. The nursing staff will record a daily schedule of treatment for individual patients. In conjunction with the charge nurse the physiotherapist can also record specific instructions on care in these records. Case histories 5.1 and 5.2 highlight the difficulties encountered in assessing dementing patients in particular.

Accidents

Accidents are more likely to occur on assessment wards than other wards. This is due to the general confusion of the new patient or possibly because of an unexpected reaction with the adjustment of drug therapy. The most common injury is a bump on the head due to a fall. The physiotherapist may then be needed to monitor mobility for a few days. The fractured neck of femur is another hazard particularly if a patient is having to walk longer distances than at home.

Pain

There is a tendency for psychiatrically trained staff to look for a mental rather than a physical origin for pain. Admission to hospital does sometimes precipitate a flare up of pain. Typical examples would be painful arthritic knees required to do more weight bearing than usual or painful shoulders due to a patient being incorrectly lifted or using a walking frame for the first time. The physiotherapist may need to persuade others when she believes a pain to have a logical physical origin or the patient's complaints may be regarded as hypochondriacal delusions.

Case History (5.7)

Two elderly ladies both suffering from depression and anxiety fell within a week of each other and each sustained a fractured neck of femur.

Each was admitted to the general hospital where one received a Thompson's prosthesis and the other a pin and plate. The ladies were duly returned to the psychiatric hospital sick bay and then to their ward when their stitches were removed.

Mrs. Z with the Thompson's prosthesis mobilised quickly on a walking frame and complained of little pain. Mrs. A with the pin and plate was slow to mobilise and complained of pain frequently. She was heavy to nurse and the junior nursing staff accused her of not trying and cited the recovery of Mrs. Z.

The physiotherapist knew that patients with a pin and plate operation for fractured neck of femur are slower to recover and experience more pain than those with a prosthesis. The physiotherapist arranged to give a short talk at the nurses' handover session. She discovered that even some of the qualified psychiatric nurses had only a very vague idea of what had happened to Mrs. Z and Mrs. A. Several had never seen an x-ray of a Thompson's prosthesis or a pin and plate *in situ* and certainly did not know why one should be more painful than the other.

Armed with more insight into Mrs. A's lack of progress the staff changed their attitude to her and became more helpful and encouraging. The psychiatrist prescribed some additional pain reducing drugs for a short period and Mrs. A was soon successfully ambulant.

Chest Infections

Patients admitted in an unkempt and malnourished state or who are severely depressed readily develop chest infections.

There is a tendency for all to be referred to the physiotherapist who quickly becomes adept at assessing those who can be helped. Toxic confusional states are a complication of chest infection making patient cooperation difficult.

The extensive use of ECT in some units for old people with depression may involve the physiotherapist with regard to some intensive chest physiotherapy prior to general anaesthetic.

Drug Induced Syndromes

The adverse side-effects of some drugs are often experienced on the psychogeriatric assessment ward as many patients may be undergoing adjustment of existing regimens or be starting new drugs. The elderly are more likely to react adversely than the young. This is referred to in more detail in Chapter 6.

Other Conditions

Any of the range of physical problems commonly affecting the elderly may of course be encountered coincidentally with a psychiatric disorder. Such patients may be expected to be rehabilitated more slowly than those who have no mental illness.

General Ward Activity

Some form of positive activity in the daily programme is encouraged for all patients. This is most likely to be provided by a day centre or the occupational therapy department. The physiotherapy department may wish to offer a regular recreational activity depending on staffing levels. It is possible that the patients left behind on the ward because of immobility or apathy are those whom the physiotherapist can most benefit by encouraging them to move.

The Ward Round

It is of vital importance that the work being done by the physiotherapist is understood by the rest of the team. It may not be necessary to attend a whole ward round if time is at a premium. The consultant is usually willing to allow the round to be arranged so that patients on whom the physiotherapist's advice is needed can be seen at a prearranged time.

In units which are entirely separate from the general hospital and its staff, the psychiatrists will expect the physiotherapist to give a strong lead in the management of minor orthopaedic problems. Similarly a close liaison will be needed between the orthopaedic surgeons at a distant general hospital and the physiotherapist. Trauma patients are frequently returned to the psychiatric unit with instructions that the physiotherapist should oversee the general physical rehabilitation without follow-up by the orthopaedic staff unless specifically requested. The ability to make splints, remove and renew plasters and make collars is essential in this context.

Physiotherapy on a Long-term Care Ward

The long-term care ward in a hospital or specialist unit is, above all, the patient's home. It is the final resting place for those who have no caring relatives or who are too disabled or difficult to be managed in the community.

The emphasis here is not on intensive rehabilitation but providing a reasonable quality of life for patients within their limitations. The majority of patients on these wards are in the late stages of senile dementia. However there are at present in long-term institutional care a number of the inmates of the old style mental hospital suffering from conditions such as chronic schizophrenia or manic depressive psychosis. Some have lived in hospital since before the Second World War and virtually know no other life. Such people may be very old indeed, in their 80s and 90s, the lack of stress they have experienced living in such sheltered communities possibly contributing to their longevity. Those with late stage neurological conditions may also be found, and sadly sometimes a misplaced young patient with for example a severe head injury or eplipsy (*see* Case History 4.9). Provision for the young chronically sick is still variable and it can be very difficult to place a young patient in a unit close to family and friends.

It is on the long-stay psychogeriatric wards that the highest proportion of untrained nursing staff are to be found. They are hard working, dedicated people in a heavy job, giving love and basic care to their patients. However, because of lack of training, many physical problems may go unnoticed. This is exacerbated by the fact that patients are unlikely to be able to communicate their needs easily. The physiotherapist is important in the maintenance of a reasonable quality of life for such patients. Regular contact with all levels of nursing staff is very important especially because they often feel that their patients are the first to lose out when resources are limited. There are two main areas of physiotherapy involvement.

The Maintenance of Mobility

The important message for all staff on these wards is that unless everyone encourages mobility, whatever their profession, then the patients will become immobile and heavy to nurse. All too often lack of time and staff lead to patients being swung on and off commodes, wheeled to the dinner table or trapped behind the tables of geriatric chairs. All this makes life easier at first but within a few weeks patients become immobile, incontinent, weak and contracted.

The physiotherapist may not be in a position to visit such a ward daily unless dealing with a specific problem. Despite this, getting to know all the patients and their likely needs is not such an insurmountable problem as it may at first seem. The ward population does not change frequently so that there is more daily continuity than on an assessment ward.

A basic plan for monitoring mobility might centre on a

weekly or twice-weekly movement session. A movement group held on the ward allows the participation of those too infirm to go out to other activities. An additional group held on a ward at a time when the most active patients are elsewhere should also be considered as it allows more time for attending to the most infirm patients.

Recreational movement sessions do not have to be regularly led by a qualified physiotherapist and a lively physiotherapy helper can make a good contribution here. Of course, the physiotherapist must put in a regular appearance at the group but not necessarily to the whole of it. The helper can be taught to pinpoint those who are less mobile or less responsive than at previous visits for follow-up by the physiotherapist. Apparatus is of limited use on a ward with dementing patients. Soft foam balls are useful but beware the patient who takes a bite out of one. Of far more use is familiar music and movement. Tapes of old-time songs and dances seem to awaken old memories and an old lady who cannot normally string two coherent words together will delightedly sing her way through a well loved waltz remembering all the words as she dances. If the less inhibited staff join in then the better the response from the patients. Children's action songs can also be popular especially if very repetitive.

During a movement group some effort should be made to get everyone, if possible, on their feet. Thus a physiotherapy helper may lead the general group while the physiotherapist with a nurse or another helper singles out individual patients. The most contracted and seemingly unresponsive patients do respond very well to rhythm. They may be seen rocking in time to music and the physiotherapist can take a cue from this by gently and rhythmically opening and closing contracted limbs. Some patients like surprisingly violent movement and only begin to smile and open their eyes when you are moving them very positively and strongly. These very contracted and demented patients often sit hunched up in a fetal position with their legs crossed and their arms tightly clenched across the chest. Once permanently contracted in this position such patients present a great problem for the nursing staff; therefore a good stretch of the limbs is most important.

Following a movement session a list of patients felt to be at risk of becoming immobile can be made. These can be the responsibility of the physiotherapy helper who will visit them regularly and check on their walking ability. A discerning helper will time her visit to coincide with the serving of dinner, for example, and see that her charges walk with her to the dinner table. In this way she ensures that patients are not pushed or lifted for speed and her efforts are more likely to be backed by the rest of the ward staff because positive help has been given at a busy time.

Walking aids and wheelchairs need regular checking on long-stay wards. They are subject to abuse by the more aggressive patients and readily become bent or unstable. Wheelchairs should be prescribed sparingly: there is something wrong on a ward in which a large number of patients are sitting around in wheelchairs and all the easy chairs are empty.

Bedsores do develop on some patients, and while these should be managed in the main by the nursing staff, the prevention of sores is an important part of the physiotherapist's role. If a sore stubbornly refuses to heal then the physiotherapist can offer one of the several available treatments as an alternative. A change in treatment regimen can often be the key to the sore beginning to heal.

Contractures

Contractures are a major problem with patients who have multi-infarct dementia. The strong spasm which they may experience does not necessarily present with a classical pattern, it may be patchy and variable. Thus a patient with a spastic arm one week may be better the next or have recurring attacks. Frequent fits create strong spasms which must be very painful.

One thing is certain, and the physiotherapist must come to terms with this—some degree of contracture cannot be avoided in certain patients. However the physiotherapist must not be complacent about this and new methods of treatment should always be investigated but however vigilant the staff, the extreme spasm which some patients suffer is very strong and sustained, nevertheless a great deal can be done to help them. Anticonvulsant drugs are available although their use may be complicated by their side-effects and interaction with other drugs. Bath time is enjoyed and is an easy time to move a patient. The nurse can be taught how best to stretch contracting limbs in the bath when the patient is warm and supported by the water.

Contracted hands are quite common in otherwise mobile patients. The claw-type hand with thumb and forefinger free and the remaining three fingers tightly clenched, nails digging into the palms is typical. Unless carefully monitored it is easy for the skin of the hand to break down as the nails dig into the palm and tinea-type (athlete's foot) fungal infections can occur. To prevent this, hand inspection at group movement sessions is essential. Graded sizes of hand rolls can be used to help to stretch a contracted hand.

Varying diameters of padded hair curlers are useful but these can only be used to effect if a patient will keep the roll in the hand. Often a patient removes the padding, or worst still tries to eat it and a roll cannot be used.

A physiotherapy helper can learn to stretch hands and inspect them regularly. An inert cream can be used to massage into the skin and keep it supple as the hand is stretched. Great care needs to be taken not to tear or bruise frail ageing skin. On a ward where a volunteer came in regularly to give manicures including the application of nail varnish great pleasure was manifested by the patients and the general standard of hand care was high.

Ward Furniture

A good range of chairs is necessary to suit all types of individuals on a long-stay ward. Advice on the style of furniture should be forthcoming from the physiotherapist.

Sometimes relatives like to buy an armchair for a patient and need help in their choice.

Other Areas of Involvement and Terminal Care

There are other areas of involvement for the physiotherapist on the long-stay ward similar to those on an assessment ward. Care of the dying is also one aspect of the work on these wards. To enable the old to die with dignity among those who care is the aim of the ward team. Patients should not be abandoned by the physiotherapist when they are being nursed terminally. Clear airways to allow ease of breathing, careful positioning for comfort and the prevention of sores are still part of the physiotherapist's responsibility. The assurance of a familiar face and a few minutes spent with an arm round the shoulders or holding a hand is not time wasted from the busy round. Anyone who has worked regularly in a unit for the chronically sick will be aware of the conflicting emotions experienced by the staff as they tend the death of someone who has suffered greatly and yet they have grown to know and love.

Continuity of care through to a peaceful end is as important for the therapist in her approach to her work as it is for the patient in his dying. This continuity must be seen by the therapist as a positive approach to the inevitability of death.

It is hard to face death frequently and if in the depths of winter a chest infection sweeps across a ward and several well loved patients die in a short space of time, all the staff need the mutual assurance that their combined efforts have provided the right atmosphere and care and no one, including the physiotherapist, has opted out of their supportive role.

Physiotherapy on the Holiday Relief Ward

Sometimes a ward is set aside as a holiday and emergency relief ward to help those caring for dementing relatives at home. The ward may offer, say, two weeks in-patient care in every six or twelve week period, to ease the burden for those at home. In addition this ward may be used to assess those with dementia rather than the acute admission ward.

Contact with the patient's relatives is the key to working on this ward. Each time a patient comes in, the relatives should have the opportunity to mention any problems at home so that some work can be done while the patient is on the ward to counter the problem. The relatives should feel free to meet or telephone the physiotherapist with appropriate problems and attend a treatment session for advice on physical problems and their care involving the patient.

One of the staff, the psychologist or the occupational therapist, may run a relative support group based on this ward. The physiotherapist should use this group as a forum to make herself known to the relatives of patients. Assuming the group meets monthly for a short talk and a social session over a cup of tea, the physiotherapist can make a point of putting in a brief appearance, perhaps at tea break time. In addition, a series of short talks by the physiotherapist, on such topics as lifting or walking aids, can be included in the programme.

It is always beneficial to make contact with relatives, and in any unit all types of wards will run coffee mornings or similar events to raise money for extra equipment. A coffee break spent at one of these events can be most useful in getting to know the relatives of patients and their problems at home.

Physiotherapy in a Day Care Setting

If a psychogeriatric day centre is attached to a hospital unit then the physiotherapist will readily be in contact with its patients and staff. If the unit is based in the community then regular contact with the physiotherapy services is less readily achieved. The development of community physiotherapy services to the elderly is patchy and psychogeriatrics is in competition with such popular areas as community services to physically handicapped children. Working with the elderly, in particular the confused elderly, often comes bottom of the list of desirable jobs.

The patients at a day centre are encouraged to be active and the atmosphere is lively and purposeful. An area may be available for the practice of daily living activities. Patients requiring specific physiotherapy can be given treatment in the physiotherapy department if the centre is hospital based. A general movement, keep fit, or exercise session can be considered. Walking aids need careful checking especially sticks which often receive the greatest wear and tear. Worn ferrules held on with sticky tape are commonplace.

An interesting new development in this field has been the travelling day hospital in the Portsmouth area which takes the day hospital team out to the patients. One day a week each of four centres is open to patients in their home area. The local community physiotherapist could make a visit to such a centre as a regular commitment when it came to the area.

Physiotherapy in Community Care

As previously stated, community physiotherapy to the mentally infirm elderly is still very disorganised in many health districts. Community physiotherapists are in short supply and with increasing demands on their services as those with mental illness and mental handicap return to the community for their basic care, the situation is likely to worsen. The physiotherapy profession as a whole needs a consistent policy on community care for the mentally ill elderly and this applies to all branches of mental illness care. In this area there is considerable scope for innovation and evaluation.

The work is eminently suitable for the mature physiotherapist returning to work after a break in service. Here is not the routine part-time job with little responsibility, but the opportunity for genuine personal initiative and development into an area of great need. The physiotherapist who can bring into community care of the mentally ill elderly not only a good general standard of physiotherapy but a mature approach to the problems of life is likely to succeed with patients, their relatives and other caring professions and achieve long-term job satisfaction.

References

1. Central Office of Information Pamphlet (1972). *Care of the Elderly in Britain*. London: Central Office of Information.
2. Dick D. H. (1982). *The Rising Tide. Developing services for mental illness in old age*. Health Advisory Service.
   Health Advisory Service
   Director: Dr P. Horrocks, Sutherland House, 29–37 Brighton Road, Sutton, Surrey SM2 5AN.
3. Kay D. W. K., Beamish P., Roth M. (1964). Old age mental disorders in Newcastle-on-Tyne. *British Journal of Psychiatry*; **110:** 146–158.
4. Sainsbury P. (1973). Suicide: opinions and facts. *Proceedings of the Royal Society of Medicine*; **66:** 579–587.
5. Consumers Association (1984). The drug treatment of senile dementia. *Drug and Therapeutics Bulletin*; **22** (25): 98.

Further Reading

Alzheimer's Disease Society (1984). *Caring for the Person with Dementia*. Alzheimer's Disease Society, Bank Buildings, Fulham Broadway, London SE6 1EP.

Arie T., ed (1981). *Health Care of the Elderly*. London: Croom Helm Ltd.

Blythe R. (1979). *The View in Winter*. Harmondsworth: Penguin Books Ltd.

Coakley D. (1982). *Establishing a Geriatric Service*. London: Croom Helm Ltd.

Meacher M. (1972). *Taken for a Ride*. Special residential homes for confused old people—a study of seperatism in social policy. Harlow: Longman.

Pitt B. (1982). *Psychogeriatrics*. Edinburgh: Churchill Livingstone.

Robb B. (1967). *Sans Everything: A case to answer*. London: Thomas Nelson & Sons.

6

Psychiatric Drugs and Their Side-effects

The physiotherapist will be both helped and hindered by the effects of psychotrophic drugs on her patients. There is much debate among doctors and their patients about the prescription of drugs for the treatment of mental illness. The importance of the major tranquillisers in the treatment of psychoses is indisputable. However, the value of drug therapy in relation to some of the milder neurotic disorders is questioned and, increasingly, ways are being sought to solve the problems of mental and physical illness with minimal prescription of drugs.[1] The prescription of psychotrophic drugs was at a peak in the mid 1970s, this is now declining and more emphasis is given to the treating of neurotic disorders by alternative methods and self help therapies. Nevertheless, drugs are an important part of the treatment of the mentally ill both in the long-term control of major illness and in the short term to give respite to the sufferer.

In this chapter drugs are referred to by their generic names. Commercial names can be identified by referring to the Monthly Index of Medical Specialties (MIMS) [2] or the British National Formulary.[3]

There are three main groups of drugs used in mental health care:

Antidepressants
Antianxiety drugs
Antipsychotic drugs.

Two other groups of drugs are also in common use:

Antiparkinsonian drugs
Anticonvulsants.

In addition there are major problems in the interactions

between the three main groups of psychotrophic drugs and other drugs which a patient may be taking. The elderly are particularly prey to the adverse side-effects of drugs. Thus, the prescription of drugs for mental illness requires great skill on the part of the medical practitioner.

Antidepressant Drugs

Table 6.1 shows the three groups of antidepressant drugs in common use, the areas of use, time taken to reach the desired effect and major side-effects. Specific points for the physiotherapist to note in treating patients taking antidepressants are discussed below.

Table 6.1 Antidepressants and their side-effects.

Drug	Main usage	Time to take effect	Side-effects
Tricyclic antidepressants	Depressive illness Anxiety states	2–4 weeks	Sedation Anticholinergic effects Postural hypotension Cardiac arrhythmias
Monoamine oxidase inhibitors	Depressive illness unresponsive to tricyclic drugs Anxiety states Phobias	2–4 weeks	Hypertensive reaction to tyramine-rich food Postural hypotension
Lithium carbonate	Manic depression Psychosis Mania	7 days	Tremor CNS disturbance Renal damage Gastric disturbance

Neurotic Depression

Physiotherapists may find themselves increasingly involved in the treatment of neurotic depression as an alternative to drug therapy. The whole area of drug therapy as a treatment for neurotic illness is being called into account. Self help and alternative therapies are increasingly in use and exercise and relaxation, combined with counselling to cope with the causes of depression, are two of the methods being studied.[4]

The Time for a Drug to Take Effect

It takes two to four weeks for the tricyclic antidepressant and the monoamine oxidase inhibitors (MAOI drugs) to reach their full effectiveness. During this period it will help if encouragement is given to persevere with a course of treatment by a physiotherapist whose patient may express disappointment with the lack of improvement. Some of the unwanted side-effects are also likely to be more prominent at the start of a course of drug therapy and gradually disappear. Provided the physiotherapist has ascertained from the patient's doctor that perseverance is what is needed, then she can encourage this in her patient helping them over a difficult period.

Postural Hypotension

Elderly patients may be particularly affected by postural hypotension which can cause sudden collapse. The effect of quick movements or change of position must be carefully considered in the planning of exercise routines. Fainting due to postural hypotension should not be confused with a faint due to an attack of panic or hyperventilation. While the elderly are most at risk from postural hypotension young patients are affected and do need to be cautioned to rest if dizzy or faint when exercising.

Anticholinergic Effects

The unpleasant effects of a dry mouth, constipation and difficulty in passing urine are the effects which are most likely to improve as the patient's body accommodates itself to the drug. The patient may also experience sweats, and sensitivity to heat and light may be affected.

Sedation

Sedation may be a nuisance to both patient and physiotherapist during treatment (*see* Case History 3.6). On the other hand, it benefits those who cannot sleep and those who are agitated. If a physiotherapist cannot effectively treat a patient because he keeps falling asleep, some discussion with medical staff may be necessary and it may be possible to alter the timing or type of drug taken to allow for effective physical treatment sessions. Antidepressants are often prescribed to be taken at night before retiring to gain maximum benefit from the sedative effect and allow maximum awareness during the day. Elderly patients are liable to become confused or agitated as a result of the sedative effects of antidepressants.

Blurred Vision

Elderly patients may have visual problems as a side-effect of taking antidepressant drugs. The patient may become aggressive, agitated and unwilling to move especially in unfamiliar surroundings. Fear, due to an inability to see, should always be considered in patients who otherwise might be branded as 'difficult' because they refuse to move.

Effects on the Heart

Tricyclic antidepressant drugs are prescribed with caution in the elderly and those with heart disease. The drugs have a direct effect on the heart and may cause congestive cardiac failure and arrhythmias. Mild oedema of the feet during a course of tricyclic drugs may be noted by the physiotherapist who, having queried this with the physician, can give the appropriate advice to the patient for reducing the oedema.

Diet

The diet of those taking MAOI drugs is of the utmost importance. A treatment card is produced by the publishers of the British National Formulary[3] and patients on these drugs should carry this or full instructions on the diet with them at all times.

The drugs cause a serious hypertensive reaction to tyramine-rich foods. The basic instructions are: Do not eat cheese, pickled herring or broad bean pods. Do not eat or drink any meat or yeast extract. Do not take any other medicine or remedy without consulting a doctor or pharmacist. Do not drink Chianti wine and only drink other alcoholic drinks in moderation.

The physiotherapist working in private practice or in the community must be alert to the restricted diet of their patients taking MAOI drugs. They should be prepared to check that patients are keeping to the diet and that they do not take additional drugs, for example to relieve a cold, without advice from their doctor.

Weight Gain

Weight gain is not listed in formularies as an unwanted side-effect of antidepressant drugs. Nevertheless, a proportion of patients, particularly those on MAOI diets do eat increased amounts of sweetened foods and gain weight. It is important to the morale of the patient as he recovers, that he looks and feels well. Careful advice on a sensible diet combined with keep fit work is a useful adjunct to looking good. For the physically disabled who grossly increase their weight the problem can cause loss of mobility.

Case History (6.1) (*see also* Case History 7.3)

Mr. *B* was a 48-year-old man. He held a managerial position in a busy firm. He was 1.89 m (6 ft) tall, formerly an active and dominant man both at home and work. Mr. *B* had become paraplegic at the age of 43.

Although Mr. *B* had been a model patient, keen, enthusiastic and determined to succeed when in the rehabilitation centre some years previously, he had never come to terms with his condition mentally. On his return home and to work the increasingly dominant role of his wife, the fears of looking foolish or attracting pity at work and the embarrassment of his teenage children, resulted in increasing depression. Mr. B was given MAOI drugs to take and had been taking them over a long period of time. Following a major row at home he took an overdose of his drugs and was admitted to an acute psychiatric ward.

The ward team discussed the importance of integrating Mr. B's psychological and optimum physical well-being. Mr. B had not stood and walked using his calipers for two years although he had left the rehabilitation centre able to walk with calipers and elbow crutches and could even negotiate stairs.

Initially hostile and uncommunicative Mr. B gradually began to respond in the physiotherapy department. He appreciated the obvious interaction between the physiotherapist and the rest of the ward team and found it a relief that the intense pressure to succeed physically he had experienced at the rehabilitation centre had given way to the feeling that neither mind nor body must be allowd to progress at the expense of the other.

Mr. B was very large and always had a packet of chocolate biscuits near at hand. He was shocked by his inability to sustain a standing position for long and was terrified of falling on the physiotherapists. The physiotherapist ascertained that Mr. B had not been weighed for over two years and he was horrified to discover he had increased his weight by nearly 16 kg to 95.25 kg. The dietician joined the team and helped Mr. B to plan his diet properly.

When Mr. B left hospital a plan of treatment was drawn up with a hospital near his place of work. Here he and his wife would be able to receive counselling sessions and he could also receive further physiotherapy on the same afternoon, in order that mental and physical care could continue to be combined and minimal time was lost from work.

Drug Dependency

The antidepressant drugs are not habit forming although mild dependency may develop in MAOI drugs if they are taken continuously for more than nine months. Symptoms of anxiety may be exhibited by patients who have been taking antidepressant drugs to good effect and fear their reduction will cause a return of the depression. Such patients may benefit from learning a relaxation technique.

Lithium Carbonate

Lithium carbonate is used prophylactically to prevent relapses in cases of manic depressive psychosis. It is also used to treat mania. This drug has relatively few side-effects and few interactions with other drugs. The prescription of the drug does have to be closely monitored because the therapeutic index is very small, that is the effective dose is very close to the toxic dose. The possible effects on the central nervous system of lithium taken in slight overdose are: drowsiness, tremor, ataxia and lack of coordination; this could affect the course of any incidental physiotherapy. Lithium in its effective dose may cause tremor which is easily treated with propranolol.

Antianxiety Drugs

There are three major groups of antianxiety drugs for use in treating the neuroses and phobias.

Benzodiazepines

Benzodiazepines have hypnotic and sedative effects.

Their extensive use for minor forms of stress is continually criticised in medical and other journals and the drugs are habit forming. The trade name Valium is as well known to the general public as to medical practitioners and is a reflection of how extensively the drug is used.

Barbiturates

The barbiturates are no longer in use as anxiolytics but may very rarely be used in cases of severe insomnia. Long-acting barbiturates are used in the treatment of epilepsy.

Propranolol

Propranolol is a beta-blocking agent which is effective in the reduction of the symptoms of palpitations, tremor, diarrhoea and the flushes which frequently accompany apprehension and anxiety.

All these drugs act quickly and a patient will feel the benefit in about 30 minutes.

Dependence on Antianxiety Drugs

The major and serious draw back of antianxiety drugs is the dependency which results if the drugs have been taken continuously, even in low doses, for periods of four months or sometimes less. In 1966 the popular song 'Mother's Little Helper'[5] cynically extolled the virtues of the little yellow pill taken to relieve stress. It has taken nearly 20 years for a significant change in attitudes. Moves are at last being made to encourage people to learn to cope with their stresses and tensions without resorting to drugs (*see* Chapter 7).

Antipsychotic Drugs (Major Tranquillisers)

Antipsychotic drugs are used in the treatment of schizophrenia, and manic depressive psychosis (Table 6.2). They may also be used to treat severe anxiety and rarely the symptoms of severe aggression or sexual deviation. There are three generic groups of drugs:

phenothiazine
butyrophenones
thioxanthenes.

Side-effects of Antipsychotic Drugs

Extrapyramidal Side-effects

It is thought that antipsychotic drugs may act by blocking

Table 6.2 Antipsychotic and antiparkinsonian drugs and their side-effects

Drug	Main usage	Time to take effect	Side-effects
Antipsychotic	Schizoprenia Manic depressive psychosis	2–7 days	Extrapyramidal symptoms (Parkinsonism) Tardive dyskinesia Anticholinergic effects Photosensitivity
Antiparkinsonism	Drug-induced parkinsonism	2–12 h	Reduction of parkinsonism Increased tardive dyskinesia Sedation Increased psychiatric disturbance

the dopamine receptors in the brain. This interference in dopaminergic transmission produces extrapyramidal symptoms. These symptoms are very like the more familiar parkinson's disease in that patients are slow, expressionless, have difficulty initiating movement and may exhibit stiffness and tremor. These symptoms are reversible on withdrawal of the drugs.

Tardive Dyskinesia

After very long administration of antipsychotic drugs irreversible side-effects similar to those of extrapyramidal symptoms are seen, but these particularly include unwanted movements of the face, mouth, upper limbs and trunk. As a result patients drool and dribble, and are unable to speak clearly and have eating difficulties. This condition is called tardive dyskinesia. Many different treatments have been tried with these unfortunate patients but few are even partly effective. The syndrome has led to greater caution in the long-term prescription of major tranquillisers.

Photosensitivity

Photosensitivity may occur as a side-effect of some antipsychotic drugs, in particular, chlorpromazine. Treatment with ultraviolet light is therefore contraindicated in patients taking these drugs. Care must be taken when these patients go out of doors especially on bright sunny days.

The Administration of Antipsychotic Drugs

Antipsychotic drugs may be administered by mouth, as suppositories or by injection. Many patients need long-term drug therapy.

This used to present problems because schizophrenic patients often defaulted and then lapsed into an acute episode of their illness. The incidence of acute attacks of schizophrenia has considerably reduced as a result of the depot injection. These injections take effect quickly and their effect lasts for two to six weeks. Patients who default from injection sessions can be followed up by a social worker or community psychiatric nurse and persuaded to attend for treatment.

Antiparkinsonian Drugs

The extrapyramidal side-effects of the antipsychotic drugs can be countered to some extent by anticholinergic drugs such as benzhexol, orphenadrine, and procyclidine (levodopa is contraindicated in drug induced parkinsonism). These drugs are not administered routinely for they in turn have side-effects (Table 6.2), and may even be abused. The following points should be considered concerning anticholinergic drugs:

The effects of the antipsychotic drugs may be reduced.
The increased effect of tardive dyskinesia produced is irreversible and therefore undesirable.
Sedation reduces the mobility of patients.
Hallucinations and other psychotic symptoms may be induced.

Physiotherapy Involvement in the Treatment of Drug Induced Extrapyramidal Symptoms

Physiotherapists are frequently asked to treat patients suffering from the side-effects of antipsychotic and antiparkinsonian drugs. No quantitative work has yet been published on the effectiveness of physiotherapy in parkinsonism and tardive dyskinesia, though it is reasonable to suppose the rate of contracture and immobility can be slowed in patients whose physical well-being is constantly monitored. Perhaps the most difficult message to convey to the ward team is that there is no way physiotherapy can cure the side-effects of antipsychotic drugs. All that can be done is to try and prevent irreversible contracture and immobility and improve mobility if drug therapy is discontinued especially in tardive dyskinesia. A positive approach to the problems is important for the morale of patients and staff. The physiotherapist can help in the following ways.

Teaching

The symptoms of extrapyramidal lesions may not be fully understood by some of the ward team, in particular student nurses, nursing helpers and non-medically biased therapists such as art or music therapists. The physiotherapist could arrange a teaching session emphasising such aspects as cog wheel rigidity, difficulty in initiating movement and the tendency to fall backwards. A discussion can be held about ways in which these problems should be countered, such as by reinforcing rhythm when walking (patient and therapist counting or singing), guiding hand to mouth for initiating of movement at the start of a meal or working on rhythmical patterns in art and music. If the staff understand the patient's movement problem then the patient is likely to be more relaxed and succeed, anxiety is known to worsen both extrapyramidal symptoms and tardive dyskinesia.

Provision of Walking Aids

Walking aids are generally a failure where the treatment of parkinsonism is concerned. The physiotherapy journals and trade magazines often have new ideas and adaptations, but so far all fall short of the ideal. There are two barriers to the successful use of a walking aid. First, the tendency to fall backwards means that as a patient lifts a walking frame up from the floor the movement causes him to tip backwards. Second, rigidity and inability to initiate movement causes the patient to shuffle and fall over his feet or rush into the frame itself before it can be moved forwards. Experiments with flexible guards at ankle level to remind the patient to lift his feet have claimed some success but mentally confused psychiatric patients are unlikely to respond to this.

Some patients are able to walk well using a rollator-type walking aid with wheels at the front and stops at the back. These frames are rather large and therefore more useful in a hospital than at home. In addition they are heavy and difficult to manoeuvre when turning round.

The only alternative is to walk with the patient enabling him to lean on a comforting arm and if necessary counting or singing to sustain the movement. Patients who have ceased drug therapy because of extrapyramidal symptoms are probably best encouraged in this way and may soon start to get about on their own as their symptoms diminish. For those with permanent disability this may be their only means of getting about for the rest of their lives. The case history that follows illustrates an extreme case of irreversible tardive dyskinesia.

Case History (6.2)

Miss *A* a woman of 67 had been an in-patient in a psychiatric hospital for many years. She suffered from manic depressive psychosis and was receiving regular medication, antipsychotic drugs in tablet form. Miss *A*'s formerly mild parkinsonism became more pronounced and it was decided to try using antiparkinsonian drugs. Initially all went well and Miss *A* seemed to improve but then she produced some quite dramatic symptoms. Her legs and arms became contracted and weak, speech deteriorated and her hands were tightly clenched. At first it was thought that this might be due to a cervical lesion as a result of arthritis in the neck but a full neurological investigation revealed that despite the delayed response, drug therapy was at fault. Miss A came to the hospital sick bay and antiparkinsonian drugs were discontinued. The physiotherapist was asked to help to try and improve Miss A's physical state.

Miss A was curled into a fetal position, she could not walk or feed herself. Her speech was very difficult to understand due to the constant writhing of her tongue. After three months of daily treatment the physiotherapist decided to consider with the ward team whether more could be achieved. Miss A could sit in a chair but still had flexion deformities at the knees and hips. She held her arms in abduction at the shoulders and this combined with flexion deformities at the elbows prevented her reaching the handles of a walking frame even with the handles raised to the maximum height. Both hands were contracted and clenched, and it was virtually impossible to cut the finger nails on her right hand.

However, by the end of nine months Miss A could walk with the aid of one person and feed herself with a spoon. Her symptoms of gross tardive dyskinesia remained and the patient needed constant monitoring to prevent a lapse into total immobility again.

The main lesson the physiotherapists learned from this extreme case was how long it was necessary to persevere with treatment to gain maximum effect and this is generally so in the treatment of the mentally ill who are slow to respond in comparison with those who have only to contend with physical illness.

Anticonvulsant Drugs

Epileptic patients have their fits suppressed by long-term medication with anticonvulsant drugs. Phenytoin, phenobarbitone, carbamazepine and sodium valproate are the major drugs of choice. These drugs often interact with each other and other drugs and therefore need careful monitoring by the medical practitioner.

Drug Interactions and Prescribing for the Elderly

The adverse effects of the interactions of psychotropic drugs with other drugs and the problems of the extreme sensitivity of the elderly to drug therapy must be carefully considered by the physiotherapist. Extreme reactions, unexpected confusion or sedation may be due to drug therapy and the appropriate medical practitioner should be consulted if in doubt, (*see* Case History 3.2).

References

1. Morris J. N. (1983). Exercise, health and medicine. *British Medical Journal*, **286:** 1597–1598.
2. Monthly Index of Medical Specialties, Medical Publications Ltd, 76 Dean Street, London W1A 1BU.
3. British National Formulary, British Medical Association, Tavistock Square, London WC1H 9JP and The Pharmaceutical Press, 1 Lambeth High Street, London SE1 7JN.
4. Pietrioni P. (1983). Can we turn a blind eye to holism? *BMA News Review*, **9,** (12): 24–25.
5. Jagger M., Richard K. (1966). *Mother's Little Helper*—A popular song. London: Essex Music International.

Further Reading

Tyrer P. J. (1982). *Drugs in Psychiatric Practice*. London: Butterworths.

7

Techniques for the Relief of Stress

Throughout this book there has been a consistent theme, namely that neurotic disorders are best treated by trying to understand, face and overcome, or come to terms with the problems causing the stress rather than the resorting to drugs. Stressful situations are a normal part of everyday life and in common with all mammals our bodies are designed to respond automatically to stress in a particular way. That response is sometimes termed the *'fight or flight reaction'* and is an involuntary reflex action designed to heighten the sensitivity of an animal when in danger or when it needs to draw on extra reserves such as when hunting for food.

Modern man still needs the fight or flight reaction to heighten his performance in everyday life. However, the pace of life in civilised society has become such, that some stress provoking situations are so frequently repeated, or continuous, that the fight or flight reaction once initiated is never counteracted and the subject continues to experience the unpleasant physical symptoms of the reaction.

Two typical examples of the initiation of illness due to stress are illustrated by Case Histories 7.1 and 7.2.

The Initiation of an Anxiety Neurosis

Case History (7.1)

Mr. *C* a double glazing salesman was 30 years old, married with two small children. His wife was expecting a third child and the couple were buying a new house on a modern estate by means of a building society mortgage. Mr. *C* earned a small basic salary but the bulk of his pay was calculated on a commission basis according to his personal sales record. A slump in the economy caused several major local employers to make economies, one factory closed and at others the staff numbers were reduced. Many people were on short time working and no one could afford the additional luxury of double glazing. Mr. *C*'s take home pay steadily fell. He could no longer afford any luxuries and he began to fear he would not be able to meet his mortgage repayments. Increasingly Mr. *C* was seen in his general practitioner's surgery. He complained of severe headaches and pains in the neck and shoulders. At other times he presented with digestive disorders complaining of indigestion and stomach pains. Mr. *C* was unable to sleep and gradually became obsessed by his many physical symptoms, convinced that he had an undiscovered physical illness.

The Initiation of a Phobia (Agoraphobia)

Case History (7.2)

Mrs. *D*, her husband, a long-distance lorry driver, and their two children, a baby and a toddler had recently been rehoused in a block of council flats some miles away from the area in which Mrs. *D* had been born and brought up. The flat was on the first floor and had no garden or balcony. Mrs. *D*'s husband was away a great deal and Mrs. *D* could not drive their car. Mrs. *D* felt lonely and isolated and the groups of teenagers with motor bikes who collected in the entrances and courtyards of the flats made her feel nervous.

Mrs. *D* struggled down the stairs with her baby, toddler and pram to go to the supermarket. The shop was crowded and impersonal. The toddler had to walk round the store, the baby sat in the trolley. The toddler kept grabbing tins and throwing them in the trolley. One tin hit the baby who started screaming. Mrs. *D* smacked the toddler who also screamed. Eventually the family joined the long check-out queue and Mrs. *D* picked a packet of sweets from the nearby stand and gave it to the toddler to pacify him. The lady behind them in the queue made a rude comment to her neighbour about modern mothers bribing their children who were uncontrollable. The baby continued to cry and Mrs. *D* began to feel the air in the supermarket was close and felt faint.

A few days later Mrs. *D* went shopping again, she tried to hold the toddler's arm as they went round the supermarket and he wriggled and screamed. Eventually the toddler started demanding sweets and Mrs. *D* remembering the comments made on the previous visit refused sweets. The little boy lay on the floor and had a tantrum, he kicked out and knocked over a pile of tins. Mrs. *D* stood embarrassed and miserable in the long queue. She felt the air oppressive and gasped for breath. She had to leave before she made an exhibition of herself. Mrs. *D* grabbed the children and rushed out of the supermarket abandoning her trolley of shopping.

Mrs. *D* made excuses when her husband came home saying the baby was feverish. She persuaded him to shop for her the following morning and he was late for work. Insidiously Mrs. *D*'s husband found himself doing more and more, it gradually dawned on him that his wife never left the flat. One day he persuaded her to come out to the shops but as soon as they reached the crowded high street she began to gasp for breath and said she was going to faint. Mrs. *D*'s husband found he was affected at work. He could not be away from home because his wife and children needed him to shop for them. Mrs. *D*'s husband went to see their general practitioner and told him what was happening.

A Revision of the Physiological Response to Stress

The physiological response to stress and the fight or flight reaction are controlled by the autonomic nervous system. The autonomic nervous system supplies involuntary muscles, secreting glands and the heart. The centres in the brain for the control of the activity of the autonomic system are in the medulla, the hypothalamus and the cerebral cortex. The hypothalamus and the limbic lobe of the cerebral cortex form the limbic system which is the higher centre of control for that part of autonomic activity particularly associated with emotional reaction.

The autonomic nervous system is subdivided into two separate nervous systems—the *sympathetic* and the *parasympathetic*. The two systems frequently act in a complementary manner thus when the activity of one system supplying an organ increases, that of the other decreases. This is effected by the quantity of the chemical transmitter released at the nerve ending. The sympathetic system emits a transmitter called *noradrenaline* and that released at parasympathetic endings is *acetylcholine*. Thus the effects produced by the sympathetic system are termed adrenergic and those by the parasympathetic system cholinergic.

Noradrenaline is also released as a hormone by the adrenal gland and its circulation in the body from this gland will augment the activity of the sympathetic system.

The Sympathetic System

The sympathetic system is activated in times of stress initiating the fight or flight mechanism and the body becomes poised for action, the pupils dilate and the mouth dries, the heart beats faster, the pace of breathing quickens and the muscles tense. The sphincter muscles close and the additional secretion of noradrenaline and adrenaline from the adrenal glands boosts and prolongs the reaction.

The Parasympathetic System

The activity of the parasympathetic system which is mainly concerned with the emptying mechanisms of the body, the secretion of gastric juices and the vasodilatation of the erectile tissue of the genitalia is usually inhibited by sudden sympathetic activity. However, in cases of extreme fear the parasympathetic system may over-react and cause sudden emptying of the bladder or diarrhoea.

During normal activity there is a delicate balance between the sympathetic and parasympathetic systems. The arrival of an appetising meal on the table stimulates the parasympathetic system into dominance and the digestive system operates.

The need for extra vigilance in crossing a busy road stimulates the activity of the sympathetic system and the body becomes alert. Each time there is an appropriate return within a short period to the balance between the systems.

What happens if the cause of the stimulation of a fight and flight reaction does not go away? Often the body adjusts to the physical side as the subject comes to terms with the problem in his mind. Learning to cope with small amounts of stress is good for body and mind, it keeps both systems alert and able to manage. However, some stimulation is so unpleasant, frequently repeated, or continuous that the level of noradrenaline in the body is maintained at a constantly high level with all the unpleasant physical sequelae. In the case of the woman who experienced the unpleasant panic attacks in the supermarket it may even be fear of the fear itself which keeps the level of noradrenline abnormally high in her body.

Physical Symptoms and Signs of Anxiety

Symptoms

It is frequently the physical symptoms of anxiety that a patient first presents to his doctor. The patient often does not recognise that there is a mental cause for his problems. Even if the patient does suspect that deep down the cause may be worry the more acceptable face of physical illness creates an unconscious blocking in the mind as to the real root of the problem. It is much easier unwittingly to express anguish, worry or fear with a physical front which others will understand, and the over-reaction of the sympathetic system conspires with the unconscious mind to perpetuate the deception. Of course, the patient really does feel pain, anyone who holds his shoulders tense for long periods will develop neck and shoulder ache, anyone whose digestive juices are not freely released will experience indigestion, anyone who breathes erractically in gasps will experience tingling in the hands and feet and faintness. The symptoms which are most frequently presented as cause for complaint are listed and a patient may concurrently exhibit several symptoms.

Headaches may radiate from the forehead down the back of the neck. The headaches may be associated with insomnia. Dizziness may also be a cause of complaint.

Blurred vision may occur partly due to dilation of the pupils, this may also be combined with dizziness.

Perpetually *dry mouth* and altered taste may accompany a more general digestive disorder.

Digestive disorders are common with feelings of nausea and indigestion as a result of reduced secretions. Ulcers, colitis and chronic constipation or diarrhoea may be the end result.

Hyperventilation and associated breathing problems may result in frequent faints. The possibility of epilepsy has to be excluded from these patients. Many physical symptoms such as tingling fingers and palpitations are associated with hyperventilation.

General *muscular aches and pains* in particular neck ache and low back pain occur. The perpetual poor posture of a patient with combined depression and anxiety heightens this type of pain.

Asthma may be exacerbated by anxiety as may disorders of the heart. Patients with acute anxiety may present with high blood pressure.

Lowered resistance to infection is also thought to be caused by the physiological effects of anxiety and such patients suffer from recurrent colds and infections. Allergies in the form of skin rashes and diseases also occur. Excessive sweating also produces skin rashes.

A distressing symptom for men is the fear of *impotence* due to an inability to maintain an erection of the penis which is governed by the parasympathetic system. This is another example of a complicated reaction in which the prime anxiety causes a physical disability which causes a secondary fear. This secondary fear then becomes the major cause of concern for the patient.

Signs

The physiotherapist is trained to observe. Much can be learned about the state of a patient's mind by observing his body language. The cover of cheerful conversation can be broken by observing restless feet or tightly gripped hands. Typical signs of tension are:

Frowning

Inability to make eye contact
Clenched teeth and tight lips
Jutting jaw
Hunched shoulders, one or both
Restless hands which fiddle with hair or tap on the table
Nail biting
Arms tightly folded or hands clenched
Perching on the front of a chair
Frequent sighs and fidgeting when waiting
Crossing and uncrossing of legs
Toe tapping.

Many people have individual quirks which they display when faced with a worry such as incessant humming or jiggling money in the pocket. The Turks have special beads, called worry beads, which they carry in their pockets for this purpose.

The Treatment of Stress Related Disorders

Consultation

The first step taken by a psychiatrist, general practitioner or psychologist when assessing a patient with an anxiety neurosis or phobia will be to listen to the patient and talk with him to reach the root of the problem and decide on a course of action. Various methods may then be used to help the patient overcome the problem.

Drug therapy in the form of antianxiety drugs and antidepressants will be used sparingly, perhaps to enable a patient to think more clearly, or gain some much needed sleep. Simple psychotherapy may then follow to help the patient recognise the root of the neurosis and either take the appropriate action to resolve the causes or try and compromise over problems which are insoluble. Patients with gross physical symptoms must understand and accept the mechanism which has created those symptoms in order to be able to overcome them. The psychiatrist may need to eliminate the possibility of various physical illnesses as the cause of physical symptoms; but great care must be taken not to overemphasise physical disability. No patient will recover properly if he still believes his physical symptoms may be caused by some undiscovered physical illness. A few patients, usually young people, whose symptoms are due to extreme difficulties in forming satisfactory relationships with others may be referred to a psychotherapist for prolonged treatment.

Behaviour Therapy

Behaviour therapy is often the treatment of choice for patients suffering from phobias. The behaviour therapist introduces a patient to a planned programme which includes repeated contacts with the situation causing the phobia. The patient is encouraged to return repeatedly to the situation causing the stress. A technique for relaxing and how to apply it in the stressful situation is also taught.

Physiotherapy Involvement in Stress Control Techniques

In the context of this book the techniques described are used with patients receiving treatment for mental disorders. The treatments are however applicable to many everyday situations with people who are not mentally ill. Increasingly, courses are advertised at colleges of adult education and businessmen's centres on stress relief techniques. The usefulness of the systems for many groups of people, from young mothers with small children to those suffering from heart disease, is now being recognised.

Physiotherapists are an ideal profession to teach stress relief techniques. Their intimate knowledge of the body and the way it works enables them to pinpoint small details which could go unnoticed. In movement therapies which encourage extremes of free movement a knowledge of what is safe and what may cause damage is important. The physiotherapist must not teach her technique in isolation but must listen to her patients and help them to apply the technique to their problems in a practical way.

Methods of Relaxation

In the same way that individual people have their own private methods of relaxing themselves, teachers of relaxation tend to develop their own method of teaching relaxation. The relaxation method preferred by a physiotherapist will depend on many variables such as her own character and preferences, the problems and responses of individual patients and the facilities available for teaching. It is best if the physiotherapist can acquaint herself with several different ways of teaching relaxation, while she may then tend to favour one method and use it predominantly, patients who do not respond can be found an alternative.

The Contrast Technique

The most widely used method of relaxation is based on the contrast technique. This method was devised by Edmund Jacobsen[1] and relaxation of the whole body is obtained by the systematic strong contraction of the muscles held in tension and their relaxation, starting at the extremities and working up to the head gradually including the whole body. The fact that this system is so widely used means that many people will have heard of it or even used it before. Thus it is a simple system to teach and the step by step routine is easily understood by patients.

This system does have its disadvantages however. It is difficult to teach patients to relax unobtrusively in tense situations if they have to clench themselves and then let go to initiate the relaxation response. In addition some patients who hold themselves very rigidly do not really let go fully after a contraction and thus never really gain that full sense of total relaxation necessary between body and mind.

The Laura Mitchell Method

Many physiotherapists prefer to teach relaxation by the method described by Laura Mitchell.[2] This method involves contracting the muscles acting as antagonists to the muscles held in tension and inducing reciprocal relaxation in the tense muscles. Thus a patient will be asked to stretch his fingers and spread his hand then stop stretching rather than clench the hand and let go as is the Jacobsen technique. Similarly, pulling the shoulders down before the command to stop pulling, is encouraged rather than lifting the shoulders. Using this method the patient has consciously to move fully out of the position of tension.

This method has much to recommend it because it is simpler to apply quickly and unobtrusively in a tense situation than the contrast method. It is easier to pull the shoulders down and stretch the hands without being noticed by others than to clench up before letting go—a more obtrusive movement. Stretching is an automatic method of relieving muscle tension.

Yoga

Yoga in its fullest context is a way of life, a Hindu system encompassing discipline of the mind and body to achieve a spiritual union of the soul with the universal spirit. Devotees of yoga in its fullest context would say that in order to achieve maximum benefit to one's way of life all aspects of yoga must be studied, each level being approached in the appropriate sequence and this would involve commitments such as becoming a vegetarian. However, the yoga systems which are popular in the West are concerned with teaching postures, which are held, while practising controlled breathing and relaxation. Some of the postures are likely to throw strain on a person's body if it is not naturally supple, and therefore the tutor must be experienced in order to avoid injury. Physiotherapists do not teach yoga in their professional capacity but should not discourage a patient's interest in the technique. A patient who is interested in yoga should be advised to go to a reputable teacher and to check with his psychiatrist that this practice may help. Local adult education centres often offer yoga as an evening class and they employ experienced teachers. Some patients comment on the fact that they once practised yoga with benefit and can be advised to re-start.

Meditation

Various forms of meditation are practised in all cultures. Prayer, perhaps with the aid of a rosary, or in the ritual form of repetitive prayers, is a means of meditation. Transcendental Meditation, which is a form of meditation taken from one of the levels of the yoga system, can be practised in isolation. The benefits of meditation as a method of calming the mind and body are recognised by the medical profession,[3] but the positive improvements which can be gained in physical and mental well-being are not universal. Meditation may be contraindicated in psychotic conditions and epilepsy because of the adverse effects it may induce, thus the advice of a medical practitioner with experience of meditation may be valuable in such cases.

Hypnosis

Hypnosis is another means by which relaxation of the body and mind can be achieved, but again the advice of a medical practitioner experienced in hypnosis may be useful.

The Alexander Technique

The Alexander Technique,[4] used as an aid to the reduction of tension, is particularly popular with solo performers such as musicians and actors. The system is based on control of the body and seeks to change muscular habits, which, through maintaining the body in undesirable positions lead to pain, strain and increased tension.

Other Methods of Relaxation

From time to time various systems of meditation and relaxation become popular and most are successful for some people. Thus it is wise to be open minded about new methods, while always ensuring that no exploitation of vulnerable people is taking place. In the context of the mental health care team the physiotherapist should always be in a position to put a patient's queries to the whole team and those with the appropriate experience can advise accordingly.

Teaching Relaxation

Setting

Relaxation should be taught in a quiet warm setting. Preferably the room should have a restful colour scheme, subdued lighting and be evenly warm but airy. A new department may be fortunate in having a sound-proofed room especially designed for relaxation though it must be remembered that a total absence of extraneous noise is not normal and may worry some people. Some interesting work has been done in the field of sensory deprivation and the heightened suggestibility of some people during a period of sensory deprivation could be an argument in favour of a fully sound-proofed room for relaxation.[5]

Comfort

The patient should be warm but not hot and be dressed comfortably without restriction. A comfortable position should be chosen in lying, half lying or supported sitting, to suit the patient. Pillows and footrests can be used for additional comfort.

Assessment

Each patient is first assessed by the physiotherapist as to

the type of relaxation programme most likely to be suitable. The patient may have positive ideas on his own problems and how he can tackle them. Physical problems may preclude a patient taking up certain postures such as lying flat where there are breathing difficulties. Postural defects should be noted as should specific aches and pains.

Understanding Relaxation

A clear understanding of the body's reactions, and the way in which relaxation will help, must be held by the patient. If the patient does not understand or accept the reasons for the treatment, he will not succeed. The physiotherapist should have prepared a simple explanation of the fight or flight mechanism and the way in which relaxation will cause a calming effect and reduce somatic symptoms.

The Aims of Relaxation

The patient should understand that there are three aims in teaching relaxation:

To reduce the effect of somatic symptoms induced by anxiety or fear

To learn a technique that will enable a prolonged period of rest without worry to be taken

To apply the same technique quickly in a situation of extreme panic or anxiety to reduce the stress of the situation.

Individual Relaxation

It is advisable for many patients to have individual relaxation tuition initially. They may subsequently join a relaxation group but they are more likely to succeed with the individual attention of a one-to-one relationship, at least at the start of treatment. The technique should be practised daily by the patient who may take several weeks to master it. During this period the patient may attend a regular relaxation group held in the physiotherapy department to reinforce his work at home. If receiving individual treatment only, then a few visits to the physiotherapist at increasing intervals of time are indicated with the proviso that the patient can telephone for an extra consultation if necessary.

Once a technique is grasped it can then be applied to particular situations. The patient should be able to use relaxation in lying, sitting and standing positions. When a patient is well versed in the feel of whole body relaxation he should start to decrease the time it takes to reach that stage. Thus when the feeling of tension or panic begins to build up in a feared situation the patient should be able to say to himself. 'Stop, pull your shoulders down, stop pulling, breath out slowly' and reduce the panic mechanism. This can be practised in a department while imagining an unpleasant situation. Subsequently it can be practised in the appropriate setting, if necessary in the company of the physiotherapist, a behaviour therapist, friend or relative.

Group Relaxation

Group relaxation sessions are popular and effective for many, not least for their social aspect. Much harm has been done to the concept of relaxation group work in some hospital wards because of their blanket application to all the patients at once. Often such groups are led by a relatively inexperienced nurse who cannot hope to benefit the individuals of such a diverse group. A relaxation group should be chosen with care remembering that tension control techniques are aimed at helping the individual.

Physiotherapists cannot expect to treat more than about ten people together and a better number is six or eight. The constitution of the group should also be flexible to allow regroupings with others or individual work with those whose temperament does not fit in. Patients should not all be expected to adopt the same posture for relaxation but ample alternatives should be available in the form of chairs, couches or cushions.

Where mixed sex groups are taught patients need to be reminded to wear suitable clothing which will not embarass them or others by revealing large expanses of flesh or enticing underwear. The excellent cheap jogging suits available in all sizes and shapes are ideal for relaxation.

The physiotherapist should start the group by allowing patients to relate to one another, perhaps briefly talking about what has happened since the last group and refreshing memories on peoples names. Newcomers need introducing and welcoming so that all are reasonably at ease. At the end of a session, time should be set aside for another brief discussion allowing people to express their opinions on the outcome of the session. The provision of an informal cup of tea at the end of a group could allow time for the physiotherapist to move among patients and pick up any individual problems.

The frequency with which a group meets is a matter for the physiotherapist to decide. Weekly sessions for six weeks might be suitable but some flexibility to suit individual needs must be allowed.

The social aspects of group relaxation are important. Patients often help one another in their problems which is why they need time to talk. However, some people cannot concentrate with others around and need the privacy of individual sessions.

Aids to Relaxation

There are a number of aids which can be used to help achieve a state of total relaxation.

Movement

Movement is a useful adjunct to achieving a relaxed body and mind. The value of a regular sporting or keep fit activity to a sedentary worker is well known. Movement can release tensions and frustrations, free stiffened limbs and help express repressed feelings and ideas. Group or individual relaxation sessions could benefit from starting with some movement work. Free work encouraging flowing movement, swinging movements and simple back mobility are useful. Patients should be aware of the difference between rigidity and floppiness and if they have had a sedentary day the movement will make the body more supple and ready to relax.

Postural Training and Lifting

Poor posture is a frequent manifestation of anxiety. Relaxed posture should be taught. Postural self-analysis using a long mirror is valuable and a patient who is taught to be self observant may himself notice that he perpetually carries one shoulder higher than another. He can then correct this himself by glancing at his reflection in a shopwindow and correcting his shoulder level until a good posture is maintained unconsciously. Poor posture as a cause of neck and backache in anxiety neurosis is common. The opportunity should be taken to remind people of the correct way to lift. Backache is exacerbated by incorrect lifting and this is then worsened due to tension (*see* Case History 3.7).

Imagery

Various forms of imagery can be used in relaxation therapy. The physiotherapist should appear calm and relaxed as an example to the patients. Above all the voice should soothe and reassure. The patients must feel confident and trust in the physiotherapist, comfortable in the atmosphere which is being created.

Visual imagery is useful as a patient fully relaxes, for example thinking of lying on a warm beach with the waves lapping or snoozing in front of an open fire.

There are some patients who find visual imagery frustrating as it conjures up scenes of things they can never have. These people may find a blotting out technique more appropriate. In this technique one word can be repeated over and over to blot out other thoughts, a calming word such as 'peace' may be used or a repeated slow count to ten.

It has already been stated that some people cannot relax in total silence and need some form of background, in these cases unobtrusive quiet music without great extremes of instrumental or tonal variation can be used as a background. Tapes of chamber music by Mozart or Vivaldi work well if played very quietly.

Breathing and Hyperventilation Syndrome

Disturbed breathing patterns are common in anxiety and phobic neurosis. The patients develop a habit of breathing in erratic gasps of different depths and the breathing is punctuated by sighs. During a panic attack the gasping becomes rapid and the patient continues overbreathing until he faints.

Some important work has recently been published on the successful treatment of hyperventilation by physiotherapy. The work has been carried out at the physiotherapy department in Papworth Hospital, Cambridge and while this hospital is for the treatment of chest and heart disease the work has a major application in the field of psychiatry.[6]

Physiologically the overbreathing causes a blowing off of excess carbon dioxide from the body. This upsets the delicate chemical balance in the body. Motor and sensory nerve systems become hyperirritable as a result of the increased alkalinity of nervous tissue when the carbon dioxide level is reduced. Physical manifestations of this range from 'pins and needles' in the extremities to numbness, dizziness, fainting, palpitations, repeated sighing, etc. Hypoxia in the brain leads to fainting which is the culmination of a panic attack associated with hyperventilation.

Patients suffering from hyperventilation syndrome can be treated successfully by a course of breathing exercises combined with relaxation therapy. These patients are taught to slow their rate of breathing to eight breaths a minute allowing their upper chest to relax down and using the diaphragm to let the abdomen swell forward on inspiration.[6]

Patients are sometimes on treatment for several months but the success of the Papworth Hospital system is well documented and worth introducing into physiotherapy departments in psychiatric hospitals.

Relaxation Tapes

Many commercial relaxation tapes are available. They are of variable quality and should only be regarded as an aid. There is a danger that a patient could only relax with the aid of a tape which precludes the use of the method in specific situations. The intervals of time taken for the routines on the tape cannot be varied and may be too short or long.

The most useful form of tape is probably one made by the therapist for that individual patient to cope with his problems. This can be used at home as a refresher but not each time the patient relaxes.

Biofeedback

A biofeedback machine is used as an aid to teach a patient how to recognise symptoms of tension. The machine's electrodes may be worn on the fingers and the machine gives signals which may be audible or visible when a change in muscle tension is appreciated. The subject then learns to modify his reaction by reducing the automatic response and therefore reducing the signal. Biofeedback machines are of some use in the treatment of agoraphobics as these people who are incarcerated in their own homes are difficult to reach. Some general practitioners teach the use of biofeedback and its application so that patients can try and help themselves.

Water

The use of water as a relaxation medium should not be forgotten. Those involved in pool therapy are well aware of the relaxation induced by the warmth and buoyancy of water. While wallowing in a warm bath before going to bed is undoubtedly relaxing, unfortunately for many patients a bath could well be an expensive luxury.

The introduction of a shallow relaxation pool in some maternity units underlines the success of water as a relaxation medium. This method pioneered by the obstetrician, Michel Odent in France is useful during prolonged labour. Women who have used the system report that the water aids relaxation following a strong contraction and gives support allowing easier mobility to the heavy body.

Swimming is an activity to be recommended to many groups of people in need of a regular physical outlet. It can be less strenuous and more relaxing than jogging but provides the same physical stimulation.

Massage and Touch

The importance of communication through touch in mental illness cannot be underestimated. Where words are impossible touch conveys all the meaning necessary. The art of massage should not be allowed to decline or fall into disrepute. The physiotherapist is licensed to touch people, the very nature of her job allows her to, people expect it. Because of this 'licence to touch' the touching of the body by a physiotherapist is unlikely to be misinterpreted by a patient.

Touch by a physiotherapist should not be tentative but supportive and confident. It should be added that the physiotherapist in a psychiatric setting should not mind being touched by others. Patients who need to be touched also need to touch and may offer a friendly cuddle or hold a hand, even kiss a cheek. This especially applies to the elderly and those living in long-stay hospital wards and they should not be snubbed for in a way the staff are all the family they have.

Massage to reduce tension can be given to individual patients in conjuction with other treatment. It is time consuming but a patient may also use the time to talk, express fears and think more clearly about problems as he relaxes.

Patients can be reminded about the importance of touch at home.

Case History (7.3) (*see also* Case History 6.1)
> Mr. *B* was the man described in case history 6.1. Following his paraplegia he and his wife were distraught at the destruction of their sex life. Mr. *B*'s wife bought books on how to cope but Mr. *B* was not ready mentally to accept the dominant role his wife needed to play in their new style relationship. Mr. *B* rebuffed his wife and their relationship deteriorated until she could hardly bear to touch him. When Mr. *B* was admitted to hospital he had not been touched in a loving way by his wife or children for nearly a year. They attended to his basic physical needs and no more. 'I don't want a great deal, I just wish my wife would cuddle me occasionally' were his words. Mr. *B* and his family agreed to participate in family therapy when he returned home and this was one of the problems they hoped to overcome.

The importance of pets in the home for those in need of physical contact is notable. Stroking a cat is very calming and mutually enjoyed by cat and owner. The rough and tumble between dog and master is good for the release of tension.

In households where one person is affected by a neurotic condition, all may suffer from the withdrawal of touch. Patients need reminding to cuddle their children. Grandchildren are especially good for a recently bereaved grandparent as the children in seeking for a kiss and a cuddle for themselves, unwittingly give comfort to one who has lost a lifelong partner.

General Advice on Lifestyle

This chapter concludes with a comment on the need some people have to assess their lifestyle. The pace of modern life is very hectic and a patient may feel totally out of control. Relaxation helps a patient to slow his pace of life. A patient may need help in analysing his lifestyle and cutting back on inessentials or reducing work load. The physiotherapist is in a good position to advise on the physical activities of the day such as driving in busy traffic, dealing with the demands of active toddlers or carrying home heavy shopping. Relaxation and the control of tension cannot be taught in isolation it must be applicable to the everyday situation.

References

1. Jacobsen E. (1938). *Progressive Relaxation*. Chicago: University of Chicago Press.
2. Mitchell L. (1977). *Simple Relaxation*. London: John Murray.
3. Fenwick P. (1983). Can we still recommend meditation? *British Medical Journal*, **287:** 1401.
4. Alexander F. M. and Maisel E. (1975). *The Alexander Technique*. London: Thames and Hudson.
5. Slade P. D. (1985). Sensory deprivation and clinical psychiatry. *British Journal of Hospital Medicine*, **32,** (5): 256–60.
6. Cluff R. A. (1984). Chronic hyperventilation and its treatment by physiotherapy: discussion paper. *Journal of the Royal Society of Medicine*, **77:** 855–862.

Further Reading

Barker S. (1979). *Alexander Technique*. New York: Harper and Row.

Bond M. R. (1979). *Pain its Nature, Analysis and Treatment*. Edinburgh: Churchill Livingstone.

Brown B. (1977). *Stress and the Art of Biofeedback*. New York: Harper and Row.

Madders J. (1979). *Stress and Relaxation*. London: Martin Dunitz Limited.

8

Working in Specialist Units

A number of highly specialised units exist which require the services of a physiotherapist. The physiotherapists working in these units are themselves involved in treating patients in very specific areas of mental illness or addiction. There may be only one or two physiotherapists with experience in these special categories in the whole of the United Kingdom. This does not necessarily mean that the specialties are adequately provided with physiotherapy services. If apprehension or ignorance results in understaffing in physiotherapy departments in general psychiatric units then there is even less likelihood of a physiotherapist applying for a post in a specialist unit.

Alcohol Related Problems and Addiction Units

Under the auspices of the Mental Health Act 1983 (*see* Chapter 1) a person may not be regarded as suffering from mental disorder solely by reason of dependency on alcohol or drugs. A patient receiving treatment for this condition should therefore be doing so voluntarily unless a specific coexisting mental disorder has warranted the placing of the patient under a Section Order. There can be little hope of curing a patient of his addiction if he does not wish to be cured or to cooperate.

In the western world the drinking of alcohol is a widely accepted social habit. Other parts of the world have different customs, thus a Moslem society, while officially banning the consumption of alcohol or cannabis, may in fact turn a blind eye to the taking of the latter. The opium producing countries of the Far East in turn have a higher number of opium addicts than in the West. The problem of nicotine addiction and its side-effects on general health, in the form of cigarette smoking, is a contentious issue. Combatting the taking of social drugs to excess, in whatever form, is further complicated by the vast amounts of money, numbers of jobs and government revenues which would be lost if their production declined.

Alcohol Related Problems

Drinking alcohol to excess is a major problem in British society. In 1978 a survey of 2000 adults in England and Wales classed 14% of men and 3% of women as heavy drinkers.[1] If a unit of alcohol is defined as the equivalent of half a pint of beer, a single measure of spirits, 125 ml of wine, or 55 ml of fortified wine, then a heavy drinker is a man who consumed more than 50 units a week or a woman who consumes more than 35 units a week. By no means all these people could be defined as alcoholic, as regular drinking increases tolerance to alcohol, nevertheless the drink may affect their lifestyle, that of those around them, and considerably increase their chances of causing a road traffic accident when driving. The term alcohol dependence is only applied to a person who exhibits physical and mental changes as a result of his dependence. His dependence is demonstrated by:

> A pathological desire for alcohol exacerbated by the ingestion of a very small dose
> Blackouts during intoxication
> Symptoms of withdrawal.

Progressive Stages of Alcohol Related Problems

Heavy drinkers classically progress through a series of stages to a state of chronic dependence.

The Social Stage

The drinker increasingly seeks out social opportunities for heavy drinking within the context of his personal life. Such drinking is particularly easy for publicans, members of the armed forces and travelling salesmen. The high rate of alcohol dependency amongst medical practitioners could be partly due to the hard drinking rugby club image often fostered in medical schools which imprints a pattern of drinking for relaxation, and becomes a method of relieving stress for the qualified doctor when faced with the burden of the many problems of his patients.

The Dependency Stage

At this stage the quantity of drink available at a social function becomes overwhelmingly important. Secret drinking to avoid withdrawal symptoms begins and feelings of guilt predominate. The drinker avoids talking about his problem unwilling to accept that he has passed the bounds of social acceptability. The recent increase in alcohol dependency amongst women is cause for concern, and at the dependency stage it is particularly easy for the housewife to buy alcohol with her shopping and secretly consume it alone at home.

Addiction

At the addiction stage the individual has lost all control over his drinking habits. The craving for drink supersedes all other matters in life. He becomes a social outcast at odds with his family and what few friends remain. He may lose his job and spend all his money on alcohol, hoarding bottles of drink and suffering tremors, cramps and fits if drink is withdrawn. The major physical problems of alcohol addiction come to the fore at this point.

Chronic Alcohol Dependence

The alcoholic has suffered permanent mental and physical damage as a result of his addiction. If his family are not supportive, he may be tramping the streets as a down and out reduced to drinking methylated spirits or he may become a permanent resident of a mental hospital.

The Treatment of Alcohol Dependence

There can be no successful treatment for alcohol dependence unless the patient acknowledges his problem and wishes to cooperate.

Psychiatric and physical assessment precede any specific treatment and this includes involving the spouse and any other relevant people together with discussion of the important contributory factors such as financial matters or stress at work.

Withdrawal of alcohol requires expert nursing and skill in order to overcome the sometimes extreme bodily reactions to withdrawal. Hospitalisation may be necessary for withdrawal of alcohol, and the patient may be prescribed a minor tranquilliser to combat withdrawal symptoms and seizures. In the long term, the drugs disulfiram and citrated calcium carbimide are used in aversion therapy. These have to be prescribed with great care because of the extremely unpleasant and dangerous side-effects if even small amounts of alcohol are taken.

Maintenance of abstinence is very difficult for alcohol dependents. Organisations such as Alcoholics Anonymous are vital to the continued abstinence of many former problem drinkers.

The Psychiatric Complications of Alcohol Abuse

Alcohol withdrawal symptoms are caused by the abrupt withdrawal of alcohol and vary in severity according to the extent of the problem.

Alcoholic tremulousness in the limbs is a sign of developing dependency

Vivid auditory and visual hallucinations may occur after several weeks of heavy drinking

Grand mal fits may occur if alcohol is withdrawn from a heavy drinker after a prolonged bout of drinking

Delerium tremens is a potentially fatal condition which can occur in chronic heavy drinkers when drink is withdrawn, such as when a patient is admitted to hospital for an operation. Hospital treatment is invariably necessary for delirium tremens.

Depression and associated anxiety states are common complications of alcohol dependence. The suicide rate is high amongst alcoholics.

The Physical Complications of Alcohol Abuse

Accidents

The largest single risk to health caused by drinking is the road traffic accident and the physiotherapist has plenty of experience in treating the subsequent injuries. Intoxication is the cause of many other accidents in the home and at work. Non-accidental injuries such as the results of baby battering and wife beating are often initiated by drunkenness.

Wernicke-Korsakoff Syndrome

This syndrome is caused by thiamine (vitamin B_1) deficiency in alcohol dependents. The nervous tissue of the cerebrum and peripheral nerves degenerates resulting in peripheral neuritis and severe memory disorders. The prognosis for full recovery, despite treatment to make up the deficiency, is poor.

Polyneuropathy

Painful polyneuritis can occur separately from that of Wernicke-Korsakoff syndrome and is probably due to malnourishment in combination with the toxic effects of alcohol.

Myopathy

Pain, tenderness and degeneration of the muscles also accompanies polyneuritis. It frequently affects the large muscles around the hips and thighs or the shoulders.

Liver Disease

Alcohol has a direct toxic effect on the liver. About 25% of alcohol dependents will develop cirrhosis of the liver over a 20-year period of drinking.

Gastrointestinal Disorders

Gastritis is a common complication of heavy drinking accounting for much absenteeism from work and progresses to more major gastrointestinal disorders. Heavy drinkers also lose their appetite and the alcohol alters the bacterial flora in their intestines, essential to proper absorption.

Chest Disease

Alcohol dependents are frequently heavy smokers. They may be malnourished and are prone to inhale vomit during blackouts and fits. All forms of chest disease are therefore common in alcoholics. Tuberculosis is found amongst vagrant alcoholics.

Alcoholic Dementia

Permanent dementia as a result of brain damage due to the direct toxic effect of alcohol on the brain is a long-term complication of alcohol dependency.

Physiotherapy in the Drinking Problem Centre

People with drinking problems may be physically unfit. They may suffer from malnourishment and vitamin deficiencies. Chest disease is common and polyneuritis and myopathies are encountered. The majority of patients will be day patients but those with serious withdrawal problems will be treated as in-patients.

General Fitness

The introduction of a major fitness programme into some alcoholic units has benefited the patients greatly and helped to alter their perspective of themselves.[2]

A proportion of patients will be generally unfit having given up all forms of physical activity in favour of drinking. If unemployed, but formerly in manual work, they may have become abruptly inactive and after treatment may be physically unfit for labouring. Others may be weak due to malnourishment or have neurological complications. Alcoholics are accident prone and may have a variety of physical injuries, often due to car accidents.

Recreational Keep Fit Work

An enjoyable recreational keep fit activity can be introduced to help patients take an interest in their bodies and use free time constructively, instead of sitting around smoking and thinking about drink. The activity chosen will be adopted to suit the unit and could be anything from football or jogging to organised keep fit classes. This need is often recognised by the patients themselves in units where such activity is not provided.

The Multigym

Some units are fortunate in having a multigym. This expensive item is without doubt the most popular activity for patients and they are strongly attracted to using it. The advantage of this apparatus is the variety of individual programmes which can be produced. Specific strengthening work can be arranged for those with particular problems. Patients enjoy keeping their own record charts and an element of friendly rivalry is an added stimulus.

Specific Physical Problems

Chest Infections

Patients at risk of fitting or inhaling vomit during withdrawal seizures need careful nursing. Those with chronic chest disease probably need routine physiotherapy during withdrawal. Subsequent chest infections also need treating.

Polyneuropathy and Myopathy

The physiotherapist will be called on to manage the mobility problems associated with these conditions. The basic concepts of positioning, prevention of contracture, skin care and regaining movement apply. Patients suffer considerable pain in these conditions and recovery may be slow and incomplete. Working with alcohol dependents can be frustrating and requires patience.

Case History (8.1)

Mr. *E* at 52 was attending a day centre for the treatment of his alcohol dependence syndrome. He was a greengrocer by trade and complained of acute bilateral pain in the shoulder muscles and tingling in the hands which prevented him from lifting boxes of fruit and vegetables. Mr. *E* was convinced he had neck trouble but a thorough medical investigation eliminated this and his shoulder pains were diagnosed as an alcoholic myopathy with neuritis in the hands.

The physiotherapist was asked to see Mr. *E* and advise him. Mr. *E* insisted he had neck trouble and wanted cervical traction. He was affable and inattentive, smelling strongly of drink. The physiotherapist noted that the main problem was pain with acute tenderness of the shoulder muscles and pins and needles in the hands. Movements and strength were good. Mr. *E*'s major worry seemed to be night pain and insomnia. Alcohol dependents do not sleep well as a complication of their condition. Mr *E* slept best in an arm chair and the physiotherapist helped him to sort out a method of supporting his head and arms on pillows to aid comfort. A check was made with Mr. *E* about his lifting methods in the shop and lifting instruction was given. Arrangements were made to see Mr. *E* a week later to see if the new sleeping position was helping.

Two days later Mr. *E* came to the physiotherapy department. He said that he was going to attend a private practitioner for cervical traction. The physiotherapist once again explained that cervical traction was contraindicated because the myopathy was caused by the patient's drinking problem and that the pain would lessen if he followed the advice he was given in the drinking problem clinic.

The physiotherapist conferred with the team on the drinking problem unit. They felt they were making little headway with

Mr. *E*, his attendance was erratic and he was not cooperative. Financially he was not bothered as his wife was running the shop.

Mr. *E* did not appear in the physiotherapy department again until three months later. He suddenly 'dropped by one morning for old times sake'. He still had tender shoulders and sleeping problems, smelt of drink and he was on the way to the races. He said he had not bothered to go back for the private treatment as it interfered with his horse racing activities.

The physiotherapist felt that although she and the rest of the team had been unsuccessful with this patient at least they still had a rapport with him. He was at risk of becoming further physically disabled as a result of his addiction and if he needed treatment in the future at least there was no barrier of bad feeling between him and the physiotherapist.

This particular case history illustrates the frustrating nature of work with addicts and the need for the physiotherapist to be able to come to terms with the inevitable failure rate.

Wernicke-Korsakoff Syndrome and Alcoholic Dementia

Patients suffering from one or both of these conditions may eventually require permanent hospitalisation. Their problems and management are similar to those of patients with senile dementia as described in Chapter 5.

An additional problem when first admitted to permanent care is the immediate withdrawal of alcohol. Since this is being done on a general psychogeriatric or long-term care ward it is particularly necessary to be aware of the problems induced by withdrawal.

Case History (8.2)

Mrs. *F* was 75 and recently widowed. She and her husband had lived abroad for most of their married life and they had developed the habit of social heavy drinking. The couple returned to England on retirement and continued to drink heavily. When the husband died Mrs. *F*'s family were totally unable to cope with her now complete incapacity to function normally.

On admission Mrs. *F* was uncoordinated, unable to speak

sensibly, feed herself or walk. The sudden cessation of alcohol caused vivid hallucinations.

The physiotherapist was asked to try and improve Mrs. *F*'s mobility and help prevent further complications. A routine of daily visits starting in the physiotherapy department and then moving later in the morning to occupational therapy were instituted.

Initial treatment sessions were frankly hilarious. Mrs. *F* suffered hallucinations of the entire department being hampered by large dogs which bounded around, and of flights of birds which made unexpected appearances. Struggling on past these hazards, with the support of two people, eventually a chair would be reached but not without much giving way of knees and cries for help. Gradually the hallucinations became less frequent the last hazard to safe walking being the desire to step high over the slightest shadow on the floor.

Mrs. *F* progressed from total disarray to being able to walk alone and sit safely. Eventually despite a permanently vague aura of not being really aware of her surroundings. Mrs. *F* settled happily and was one of the few people on her ward who was always provided with a daily newspaper and could briefly comment on the headlines.

Injury

Patients may be admitted as a direct result of physical injury. More frequently they may present with an injury of recent origin which was inadequately treated due to the patient's lack of motivation and inability to keep appointments as a result of their addiction. Such patients need particularly close supervision and encouragement to regain their physical ability. A resulting deformity or handicap after an accident only serves to compound the difficulties of staying sober once dried out especially if the problem prevents the patient working again or he is obviously disfigured.

Drug Addiction

Drug addiction is rapidly increasing in the United Kingdom. The problem is particularly affecting young unemployed people. The rise of long-term unemployment in the young and the increased availability of cheap opium illegally imported from Pakistan are two major factors contributing to this.

The main groups of drugs to which people may become addicted are:

Opiates, for example, morphine, diamorphine (heroin), and synthetic equivalents
Barbiturates.

Other drugs which are illegally used include lysergic acid diethylamide (LSD), amphetamines, cocaine, and cannabis.

The prescription of addictive drugs is controlled in the United Kingdom by the Misuse of Drugs Act of 1971 and the Misuse of Drugs (Notification of and Supply to Addicts) Regulations of 1973. Only specified medical practitioners holding a licence from the Home Secretary may prescribe morphine and cocaine to addicts. Other practitioners must refer addicts to treatment centres. Treatment centres for drug addicts are few and far between in the United Kingdom and this situation is under review in view of the increasing number of addicts.

Drugs of addiction have a profound affect on the function of the central nervous system. Addicts eventually become totally physically dependent, emaciated and sick, only caring for their next dose. Many die young and in appalling physical misery. Those able to withstand the rigors of withdrawal with its unpleasant physical sequelae will emerge physically frail and prone to infection.

If new centres are set up for the treatment of drug addicts then there is a case for appointing physiotherapists to help to improve the physical rehabilitation of this group along the lines of those in units for the treatment of drinking problems.

Glue and Solvent Sniffing

A new phenomenon has arisen among older children and young adults, that of glue and solvent sniffing. Glues containing solvents such as toluene and other chemical solvents are bought and put in a plastic bag. This is placed over the nose and mouth and inhaled. The effect is similar to getting drunk on alcohol and the side-effects are the same. The following case illustrates the way in which a physiotherapist became involved with the side-effects of glue sniffing.

Case History (8.3)

At the age of 19 Mr. *G* a quiet withdrawn young man had been involved in glue sniffing for some years. He was receiving treatment as an in-patient.

Mr. *G* had developed a myopathy and peripheral neuritis. His right arm hung loosely by his side, shoulder dropped with weakened muscles, elbow weak and hand muscles wasted with a complete absence of opposition in the thumb; pain and tingling sensations were present. Mr. *G* was receiving vitamin B_1 therapy and was involved in group therapy as he tried to overcome his problems.

A daily visit to the physiotherapy department became part of the routine and passive movements to the hand which was in danger of becoming permanently contracted were followed by active work. The long mirror was used to help correct posture and soon shoulder and elbow began to return to normal with the appropriate exercise. The hand was a greater problem, while some power returned to the small muscles, opposition was stubbornly absent and remained so when Mr. *G* was discharged to his home in another area. The appropriate referrals were made but it was feared the hand might be permanently damaged.

Forensic Psychiatry

Forensic psychiatry involves the assessment of individuals whose mental condition has contributed to their involvement in criminal acts or violence towards themselves or others, and the care and treatment of those whose continuing state of mind causes them to be particularly dangerous. The majority of these patients have come into psychiatric care through the courts of law. Despite the provisions of the new Mental Health Act of 1983 there is considerable disquiet about the provisions for mentally abnormal offenders and it is generally felt that many individuals are languishing in prison when they would be better placed under the care of a psychiatrist. The courts may at present apply the act in the following ways.

Remand

An individual may be remanded to hospital for assessment or treatment prior to trial or sentence according to the type of court.

Interim Hospital Order

A person convicted of an imprisonable offence (other than murder) may be placed under an interim hospital order by the court for further assessment of his suitability for treatment.

Hospital Order

Section 37 is used for the compulsory admission to hospital of convicted offenders (other than murderers) suffering from one of the four forms of mental disorder described under the Mental Health Act of 1983 (Chapter 1).

Hospital Order with Restriction Order

Under Section 41 of the Mental Health Act of 1983 the individual may be placed under a restriction order 'to protect the public from serious harm'. This order prevents the individual from being discharged or transferred without the consent of the Home Secretary.

Not all patients who come under the care of a forensic psychiatrist are offenders. Some are admitted for treatment in forensic units because their potential for violence or antisocial behaviour cannot be contained in an ordinary psychiatric hospital.

Mental Illness Contributing to Crime

Depression and Mania

The extremes of these two disorders can contribute to criminal acts. Severe depression can result in delusions perhaps causing an individual to kill his children because of his assessment of the hopelessness of his situation or the state of the world. A fit of mania is more likely to result in grandiose ideas and lack of judgement. Borrowing large amounts of money under false pretences might by a typical misdemeanour.

Schizophrenia

Serious crimes committed by schizophrenics are rare but often receive inordinate publicity because of their extreme nature. A schizophrenic who commits a violent act is most commonly motivated by extreme delusions of persecution. Delusions of infidelity or jealousy also feature in violence perpetrated by schizophrenics.

Psychopathy

The Mental Health Act of 1983 describes a psychopathic disorder as 'a persistent disorder or disability of the mind (which may include mental impairment) resulting in abnormally aggressive or seriously irresponsible conduct on the part of that person'. Two prominent traits occur in the psychopath.

1 There is an inability to feel love or affection towards others. This inability to relate emotionally to others is often recognised as a failing in himself by the psychopath and for some it seems to stem from repetitive rejection and lack of love from others in childhood.

2 The second trait is that of total self-interest and a desire for instant gratification of personal desires irrespective of others. Thus the psychopath will take what he wants whenever he wants it, if necessary using violence to achieve his ends. He feels no remorse or guilt for what he does because he feels no concern for others.

Psychopathic behaviour is, in many cases, not amenable to treatment and dangerous psychopaths have to be compulsorily detained under a restriction order if they have committed a violent crime. Punishment is useless, the psychopath rarely relates a punishment to his behaviour and if punishment is given in retrospect this may only incite further violence. Sedatives are of little value but some hospital units are claiming success with long-term group therapy between groups of psychopaths.

A small number of psychopaths commit violent crimes of a sexual nature. Those convicted of this type of crime become notorious because of the resultant publicity. Treatment by psychotherapy for those convicted of violent crimes of a sexual nature has yielded poor results. Behaviour methods may prove more successful. Hormone therapy for men raises ethical questions because of the feminising side-effects of the drugs.

Mental Impairment (Mental Handicap)

The stress of daily life can be great for those of normal intelligence therefore it must be even greater for those who are mentally impaired. A small proportion of mentally impaired people react with violence to stressful situations because of their inability to communicate or solve a problem. Sexual offences, in particular indecent exposure, are more common in the mentally impaired than in the general population. Some of the more unsavoury offences involving young children may be committed by the mentally impaired man because of his inability to make satisfactory relationships with women. Arson is another crime which is frequently linked to mental impairment.

Considerable difficulty is experienced in nursing a

violent, mentally impaired person who is prone to self mutilation.

Units for the Treatment of Forensic Patients

In the United Kingdom patients needing treatment in secure conditions are largely cared for in two types of unit, although some hospitals may have their own secure wards.

The Regional Secure Unit

The regional secure units sometimes called regional forensic units, are a new concept. These units are in the process of being established to serve the various individual health regions. They are intended for patients who do not require treatment in the conditions of security provided at the special hospitals but who cannot be managed in ordinary psychiatric hospitals. Patients are not expected to spend years in these units and any who have not progressed out of the unit within two years would be considered for admission to a special hospital. Conversely the units may be used as a stepping off point for a special hospital patient as a start towards release into his local community. Many secure unit patients are detained there through the courts of law while others are referred individually by hospitals in the appropriate region. These units are often built in the grounds of an old psychiatric hospital but enclosed within an area of security fencing. Some staff may work entirely within the secure unit while others such as physiotherapists may work partly in the secure unit and partly in the general psychiatric hospital.

Some psychiatrists are disturbed about the introduction of the new secure units believing that they herald a return to increased custodial care and are therefore a retrograde step in the care of the mentally ill.

The Special Hospital

The special hospitals are financed by The Department of

Health and Social Security and are under the jurisdiction of The Secretary of State for Health and Social Security. About 60% of patients are detained in these hospitals under Section 41 of the Mental Health Act of 1983. The security systems in these hospitals are very extensive. The nurses wear uniforms indistinguishable from prison officers uniforms and mainly belong to the Prison Officers' Association rather than the nurses' associations.

Some patients are detained in these hospitals for many years, sometimes a lifetime, and while every effort is given to rehabilitation and final discharge, for some it is impossible. Murder, arson and violent sexual assault are common reasons for detention in special hospitals. Such hospitals house workshops, recreational facilities and education facilities within their walls in order to provide as varied and purposeful a lifestyle as possible for the patients. About two-thirds of special hospital patients are under 40 years old. The annual discharge rate is about 25% and just over half of these patients are transferred to ordinary psychiatric hospitals.

The decision to send a person to a special hospital does not set a time limit on how long he or she stays there as distinct from a prison sentence.

Prisons

Physiotherapy in prisons has not been discussed in this book. Physiotherapists who work in prisons will be well aware of the poor mental state of a number of their patients and many disturbed prisoners should possibly be in special hospitals rather than prisons. Some readers may feel there is little difference, but the difference should be in the aims and the attitudes of the carers. A special hospital is primarily a hospital and prison is a punishment. It has already been stated that psychopaths do not relate to punishment. Prisons rarely provide purposeful long-term care or rehabilitation. The prison population in the United Kingdom is the highest in Western Europe and numbers of prisoners are increasing rather than decreasing.

The Management of Violence in Secure Units and Special Hospitals

All psychiatric hospitals issue guidelines on the management of violence and the team members of each unit should be fully aware of the team policies on violence and how to react. Extreme precautions are not normally necessary but some in-service instruction should be given on how to talk to aggressive patients, the policy on physical restraint and sedation, and how to summon help. The policies that follow are those in use in the secure units and special hospitals in the United Kingdom and would most certainly not be advocated in a general psychiatric hospital. Policies may vary in other countries.

Regular staff carry keys on a long leather thong attached at the waist. The key ring may also have a whistle on it to summon help. All doors are locked and either self lock or must be locked after passing through.

Alarm buzzers are situated on the walls of individual sections of the units.

If the telephone is knocked off the hook for more than a given number of seconds an alarm is set off.

Individual members of staff may not be left alone with patients. At least one other member of staff should be present at all times.

Potential weapons must not be left lying around on wards, and staff who routinely carry equipment such as scissors must not do so in secure units.

Violent incidents must always be discussed by the ward team. Continual appraisal of management and handling techniques may reveal a way of reducing the danger of further violence. Staff too need to be able to discuss frankly their fears and need particular help if they have mishandled an incident.

Some units use seclusion or 'time out' techniques for violent behaviour where a patient is isolated in a single room for a period to calm down. Rarely, in cases of extreme self inflicted violence, perhaps if a patient continually rips open a stitched wound a nylon strait suit may be used.

Nursing staff at the special hospitals are trained in a method of restraining a violent patient involving a team of three people one of whom guards the patient's head during the incident. This system reduces the risk of physical injury to the patient and staff. Intramuscular injection of a sedative may also be used.

The Prevention of Violence in the Physiotherapy Department

In a secure situation the physiotherapist and her staff must be fully acquainted with the policy on violence in her unit. The physiotherapy department houses, without doubt, the potential for violence with its physical equipment, such as sticks, crutches and weights. This is a hazard if it is left lying about and therefore it should be safely locked in store cupboards. Patients usually enjoy physiotherapy and therefore there is a stimulus to behave, but the following points should be remembered.

Psychopaths hate waiting and readily become frustrated, therefore work loads should be adjusted to prevent crowding or waiting for apparatus.

Schizophrenics suffering from delusions of persecution must not be allowed to confuse physiotherapy with persecution. Treatment may need to be delayed if this is likely to happen despite the risk of a less satisfactory physical outcome. Nursing staff will be quick to advise on a patient's mental condition if it is considered to be particularly disturbed.

The issue of crutches and walking sticks is to be discouraged because of their potential use as a weapon. Walking frames are less of a hazard. It is difficult to stand on one leg and hit out with a walking frame. In particular, in secure situations, the ratio of nurses to patients is high and therefore there are usually adequate numbers of staff to walk with unstable patients and this is probably the best procedure rather than issuing crutches.

Physiotherapy in Forensic Psychiatry

To the reader without experience of working with forensic patients the preceding paragraphs may have made grim reading. It must however be remembered that forensic patients present an extreme of acceptable behaviour and therefore the units for their treatment are relatively few in comparison with most psychiatric patients.

Those with experience in forensic care find it interesting and rewarding. There is a greater awareness among all staff of the need for physical outlets for the body perhaps because of the daily reminders of compulsory confinement —locked doors and escorts. There is a bonus for the physiotherapist in that Regional and Department of Health and Social Security funds are available in secure units, and equipment and staffing levels are likely to be better than in an ordinary psychiatric department. Nurse escorts always accompany patients and are therefore a captive audience themselves, quick to lend a hand and interested to learn and watch the treatment of individual patients. The standards of nursing care are high and nursing helpers are unlikely to be employed therefore the physiotherapist is less likely to be frustrated by the inadequacies of poor funding levels and untrained staff.

The Treatment of Staff

It is particularly important that the staff in forensic units have ready access to physiotherapy. Violent incidents can produce trauma which is best dealt with promptly. The physiotherapist with some knowledge of the immediate treatments of the type used in treating sports injuries will find the techniques invaluable for both staff and patients. One physiotherapist working in a regional secure unit ensures that ice packs are always available in the freezer compartment of each ward refrigerator and an ultrasound machine is particularly useful as part of the basic equipment. Some units are very isolated and staff needing physiotherapy would lose much time from work travelling to distant general hospitals for treatment. The ability to provide a treatment service for staff undoubtedly improves the physiotherapists working relationship with other hospital departments and is particularly important for its immediate availability in forensic units.

Physiotherapy in Regional Secure Units

The regional secure units house a population of young active adult patients of both sexes. Between them the patients harbour a large quantity of physical energy in a confined space. There is a need to make provision for the release of this energy in a purposeful way, and this helps to prevent the occurrence of violence. The secure units are built with the following facilities which can be utilised for physical activities:

An outside recreational area
An indoor gymnasium
A multigym (available in most units)
Ward day rooms
Individual treatment rooms.

The physiotherapist will be expected to be an integral member of the treatment team and attend ward meetings, and her treatment sessions will be integrated into the overall plan for the unit. The physical programme will vary from unit to unit but should cover the following areas.

Physical Recreation

A varied programme of recreational activities can be introduced aimed at combining purposeful use of recreational time with maintaining and improving fitness in an enjoyable situation. Activities may be biased towards the needs of different groups from day to day. Team work is especially important as many of the patients have great difficulty in relating to others. Wherever possible outdoor activities should be encouraged because of the physical confinement of the patients. Natural sunlight is especially valuable because many patients choose stodgy diets and they become pasty faced and spotty but care must be taken with patients taking chlorpromazine who may be photosensitive. Smoking habits are heavy and the chance to get outside for fresh air and to expand the lungs is important.

Individual Fitness Programmes

Individual patients can be helped towards general fitness with their own fitness programme. This is where the multigym is invaluable; some secure unit staff have been known to express the worry that the use of the multigym would make patients too strong to handle. Such worries must come out in staff discussions and staff should understand that the multigym programme is used constructively to maintain patients at a level of physical well-being suitable for life in the community and any future occupation which they may be considering. If staff are worried about the fitness of patients in relation to themselves, then maybe a lunchtime fitness programme for staff is needed. Once again multigym circuits are tremendously popular and afford a maximum of activities in a comparatively small area.

Incidental Treatments

Some individual treatments may be required. As the patients are young, few will have chronic conditions. The complications of trauma are the most likely to need individual treatment by the physiotherapist.

Relaxation

Relaxation is less helpful in the severely disturbed patient than in neurotic patients. Secure unit patients find it difficult to concentrate for long periods and patients selected for relaxation therapy may only be able to relax for short sessions.

Physiotherapy in Special Hospitals

The medical directors of the special hospitals have been reassessing the aims and the role of these hospitals, no longer do they present a purely custodial image but progressive work goes on within their walls to rehabilitate and discharge as many patients as possible. For those who cannot be helped to freedom, increasingly wider opportunities are being offered within the hospitals.

In a special hospital, physical activities may be provided by several groups of professionals and because of the large size of the hospital and the poor physiotherapy staffing levels the physiotherapist will probably be providing an immediate service to the physically ill and the staff, and may have difficulty covering all the work required.

The physiotherapist based in a special hospital works across the divide between mental illness and mental impairment (handicap), about 30% of special hospital patients have some form of mental impairment. Most do not exhibit the gross problems of combined physical and mental handicap encountered in centres for mentally handicapped patients. These patients are on the whole physically able but potentially violent or sexually deviant. Some may have severe epilepsy and others repeatedly mutilate themselves. The physiotherapist in this context needs to educate herself in the problems of mental impairment (handicap).

Recreational Physical Activity

Nursing staff are often involved in the provision of physical recreation. The hospital will have traditional recreational facilities such as football pitches. A full-size swimming pool may be available and in frequent use. Each ward has its own enclosed recreational area, sometimes two in order to separate patients who annoy one another. Wards which house mentally impaired patients may have a playground area with swings, slides and climbing apparatus. At present there is little opportunity for the physiotherapist to be involved, but the potential is there.

Fitness Programme

A separately appointed remedial gymnast is likely to be involved in the maintenance of an overall fitness programme for the hospital and will have traditional gymnasium facilities for a base. In common with much work in psychiatry the role of the remedial gymnast and the physiotherapist is interchangeable and past traditions often govern appointments. The merger of these two professions in the United Kingdom in the near future will correct this anomaly.

Specific Physiotherapy

The physiotherapist is most likely to be providing a service from a traditional department dealing with individual problems in a traditional manner. There is likly to be an emphasis on the treatment of trauma as a result of violence.

The Department
Patients will be escorted to the department from their wards by two nurse escorts. These escorts wait during treatment sessions and are on hand if problems arise. A comfortable waiting area for staff close to the treatment area is necessary and escorts willingly help the physiotherapist if required. If a patient is particularly disturbed then nursing staff will telephone cancelling treatment and the physiotherapist may then visit the patient on the ward.

The Wards
The majority of patients are out at work in workshops, learning new skills or at educational and recreational groups. The temporarily severely disturbed or physically ill will remain. Telephoning the ward before a visit is advisable to avoid arriving at an inconvenient time when provision of an escort might be difficult. Nursing staff should be encouraged to discuss the physical problems of their patients and the physiotherapist will give direct advice and help. In special hospitals there are no mixed sex wards although patients of both sexes meet for socials.

Wards will be graded accordingly to the state of mental disturbance of the patients. The hospitals have sick bays for those needing special physical nursing care and here the physiotherapist may be needed regularly.

General Physiotherapy
The general physiotherapy needed is similar to that in any unit for the chronically mentally ill. Neurological problems, drug induced syndromes, the problems of ageing and incidental physical disability are frequently encountered.

Trauma and Self-Inflicted Injury
Every precaution is taken to prevent patients injuring themselves or others. Nevertheless, the physiotherapist will be needed to rehabilitate those who have suffered traumatic injury. Head injuries, severed nerves and tendons, sprains and dislocations all occur during disturbances. If the patient has inflicted the injury upon himself he may subsequently interfere with the healing process by re-opening or dirtying a wound with its attendant risk of infection, scarring and deformity. The immediate treatment of staff who have suffered physical injury has been discussed previously.

Ward Class Work
A number of wards house elderly patients whose behaviour is such that they are still unable to live outside the hospital. Recreational keep fit work of the ward class type is welcomed on these wards if the physiotherapist has sufficient time to offer this service.

General Comment

It is difficult to convey a feeling of hope and purposeful activity when describing the problems of forensic patients. To counter this the author here includes a personal note, that during the course of her researches, her visit to the physiotherapy department of a special hospital was one of the most interesting and rewarding parts of her work. The cheerful, relaxed atmosphere of the physiotherapy department and the high standard of care in the hospital wards and departments was impressive. The less stringent financial constraints on hospital expenditure enabled high staffing levels and allowed time for good interdisciplinary involvement. It is without doubt a rewarding area for specialisation.

Other Specialist Units

Brief mention is made in this section of some other types of specialist units and their aims in which a physiotherapist may be involved.

Adolescent Units

Adolescence is a disturbing time of life and adjustment to adult life is not always smooth. A minority of mentally ill adolescents suffer specific acute psychiatric disorders. The majority of those who need psychiatric advice suffer from disorders of mood or behaviour which may be due to problems at school or work, or relating to friendships. Most often the problem has its roots in family relationships and attitudes. Wherever possible an adolescent is treated in the community in the context of his home and circumstances, and in conjunction with his family.

Hospital units for the treatment of adolescents are staffed by highly motivated nurses, often very casual in their dress and specialists at creating a good rapport with their young charges who may be very antiestablishment. A few physiotherapists work with disturbed adolescents providing fitness activities suitable to the age group which are fun and in particular promote teamwork and communication. Glue sniffing and drug taking may result in physical disability which the physiotherapist will need to treat.

Mother and Baby Units

Some hospitals make provision for the care of a mentally ill mother with her young baby. The mother is most likely to be suffering from severe puerperal depression or psychosis. If the mother has to be separated from her baby because of lack of suitable accommodation then the already damaged bond between mother and baby will be worsened (*see* Case History 3.5). A mother and baby unit tries to help to prevent this separation. If the mother has only recently given birth then she may need postnatal physiotherapy and back care instruction. This can only be done in the context of the mental condition and may not be possible until the mother's mental state is receptive.

Behavioural Units

Many behavioural units practise a strict regimen based on a token economy system or reward system. Such units have claimed success in the treatment of severely disturbed adolescents and patients with head injuries. Good behaviour is rewarded with tokens or privileges and bad behaviour punished by 'time out' (banishment from the activity for a set period of time) or withdrawal of privileges. Patients are given a personal schedule to which they have to work and may even be required to buy their next meal with tokens which they have earned by meeting the appropriate targets. The meal is missed if they have inadequate tokens. Physiotherapy received by patients on such a unit will count for tokens towards privileges. The staffing levels on such a unit need to be very high for it to work properly.

Neuropsychiatric Units

The physician in charge of a neuropsychiatric unit is a specialist in differentiating between neurological disorder and mental illness. The work largely involves the diagnosis and treatment of epilepsy and defining the cause of fits, which may be due to epilepsy or be hysterical. Some of the physical problems of epilepsy are discussed in Chapter 4.

Children's Units

Psychosomatic responses to stress are common in children who may not be mature enough to express their problems verbally. Children are usually treated in the community in the context of their family situation. Physiotherapists specialising in paediatric work are more likely to encounter disturbed children in their work than those involved in psychiatry. Some physical problems in children are likely to cause psychological problems such as, head injury, hyperactivity and chronic illness. Mentally handicapped children react poorly to stressful situations and some illnesses such as childhood asthma have strong psychological links.

References

1. Wilson P. (1980). *Drinking in England and Wales*. London: HMSO.
2. Morris P. (1984). Physical fitness keeps the bottle at bay. *Remedial Therapist*, **8:** 2.

Further Reading

Edwards G. (1982). *The Treatment of Drinking Problems*. Grant McIntyre Ltd, 90–91 Great Russell Street, London NC1B 3PY.

Trick K. L. K., Tennent T. G. (1981). *Forensic Psychiatry. An Introductory Text*. London: Pitman Books Limited.

Boynton J. (1980). *Report of the Review of Rampton Hospital*. London: HMSO CMND 8073.

9

The Physiotherapy Department and its Management in a Mental Health Care Setting

In common with all professions the physiotherapist needs a base from which to work. The nature of physical therapy and the type of equipment utilised amount to a need for space to move freely and in safety. Concepts of the necessary requirements for a physiotherapist in a mental health care setting vary greatly. Some physiotherapists are obliged to work from what is virtually a small storage cupboard and others are fortunate in having modern purpose-built units. The departments suggested are modestly equipped and realistic in their requirements and many departments manage well on less. In psychiatry, in particular, withdrawal into an isolated department can be at the expense of psychiatric team relationships. It is of great value to see and be seen by the other professions. Sharing a treatment or recreation room with others may mean the effort of working out a timetable for users, but can also lead to profitable interprofessional groups such as a combined music therapy and movement group or joint occupational therapy and physiotherapy social sing-along and dance groups. Where departments and staff numbers are small such interdisciplinary combinations can be most successful.

Old Victorian hospitals have many under-used rooms and often have a large hall with a stage. This hall is frequently large enough to mark out an indoor games court and will have a high ceiling which is an advantage in racket or volley ball games.

The Atmosphere of a Department

A cheerful welcoming atmosphere is important. Pictures of interest on the walls, and posters are good talking points. An informal corner with easy chairs where a relative can sit or a patient in tears can be comforted with a cup of tea is desirable. While one cannot hold permanent open house, old patients expect to drop in with progress reports and staff may come for advice, so that, where possible, callers should not be discouraged. Communication is what much of mental health care is about.

Uniform

Uniform is still a contentious issue in many units and its use can cause considerable hostility, not least amongst non-uniformed members of staff. On the whole, acute mental illness units discourage the use of staff uniforms because of the barriers they create between patients and staff. This is especially so in units caring for adolescents. In long-stay psychiatric wards where patients are basically in their permanent home, staff may not wear uniform in order to create a more homely and casual atmosphere. Staff are expected to set a reasonable standard of dress as an example to patients who are being rehabilitated on chronic wards.

Psychogeriatric units are more likely to be run by uniformed staff. This is because confused patients are difficult to nurse in ordinary clothes. Also dementing patients often respond more readily to the ministrations of someone tangibly recognisable as a 'nurse' rather than someone in ordinary clothes who might be another confused patient.

Physiotherapists are often very reluctant to practise without a formal uniform. The reason for this is practical, as the job involves much activity and because the uniform acts as a reminder to the patient that the close physical contact he may experience from the therapist is not a sexual contact. However, there are acceptable forms of casual dress which are most appropriate for work in non-uniform units, such as trousers, sports shirt and colourful tank top or a jogging suit and training shoes. One does not become any less professional but perhaps more approachable for some patients and more acceptable to other members of staff.

Sensitivity Groups

The interprofessional relationships between members of staff in a psychiatric team should be good. Some units run staff sensitivity groups where team members of various professions can come together to air their problems and frustrations in relation to one another. Such groups can be very helpful to promoting good team relationships. Sensitivity groups are especially important for those leading group psychotherapy sessions; those involved in psychotherapy need themselves to be in touch with a trained analyst so that their own emotional ideas and reactions are not allowed to affect the patient. Ideally, all such groups should be supervised.

If a physiotherapist is closely involved in a specialist team such as on an acute ward, in a secure unit, or a unit for disturbed adolescents then she should consider making time to attend the staff sensitivity group for that unit.

The General Department

The basic minimum requirements for a physiotherapy department in a psychiatric setting are one large space for multipurpose use and a quiet room.[1] With this as the basis for development, the best of modern equipment should be provided, for the mentally ill should not have to make do with anything less than any other patients. The fully equipped modern department will include the following areas:

Large activity area (gymnasium)
Treatment area
Individual treatment room
Office/staff room
Toilet facilities
Informal area
Store.

In addition the physiotherapists should expect to make full use of any other recreational facilities provided on site such as a swimming pool or outdoor sports facilities. Community sports facilities such as sports halls are also available for use in some areas and regular visits can be organised.

Large Activity Area

This area should be large enough for group activity, group relaxation and individual remedial work. It should be light and airy preferably with access to the grounds for use during fine weather. As much small games equipment as possible can be collected over a period of time. This ensures that group work does not become boring and repetitive. Games that can be played solo are also useful, such as swingball. Portable stands and bases for netball posts and similar games ensure that best use can be made of both outdoor and indoor facilities. Typical equipment which might be considered would be:

A multigym which without doubt would be the most popular and versatile item for patients to use
Static bicycle, rowing machine and similar equipment
Indoor games such as badminton, indoor hockey and ball games
Relaxation equipment, mats, pillows and sag bags
A tape recorder and music for activity work and blank tapes for making individual relaxation tapes
Remedial equipment such as parallel bars, wall bars, stools and weight lifting equipment
Portable long mirror

Small musical instruments such as tambourines and shakers for combined music and movement activities.

The Treatment Area

The treatment area should allow room for several patients in curtained cubicles for privacy. Electrical equipment should not be displayed too prominently as it may disturb patients with schizophrenia. The area can be equipped along the lines of any small modern department with variable height and width plinths and a variety of chairs and stools.

The equipment chosen should reflect the type of condition most likely to be met in this department: soft tissue injuries are common as is chest disease, especially in the winter.

The department needs equipment for the relief of pain and the reduction of inflammation. An ultrasound machine and ice are likely to prove most useful. The addition of an Inferential Therapy unit or one of the many other types of machine using electrical currents of various types for the relief of pain can be considered. The infra-red lamp and the wax bath are still much appreciated by elderly patients who come to the department cold and stiff in the winter. The older hospitals have cold draughty corridors and even in summer some elderly patients need to be warmed up before treatment. The confused elderly may appreciate the application of a flexible heat pack to a painful area. Such a pack can be touched and felt and more readily understood than a machine. Likewise a radiant heat lamp with a warm glowing light is similarly useful (*see* Case History 5.2).

For the treatment of chest conditions a suitable adjustable plinth is important for effective postural drainage.

Activity equipment in the treatment area should include equipment for hand and foot exercises, weight lifting equipment and walking aids. A tilt table or standing frame can be used in the rehabilitation of the frail elderly or debilitated patient.

Some physiotherapy departments are now equipped with a sun bed cubicle. Some patients, particularly the younger, long-term patients, appear to receive a boost to the moral when they look sun tanned. Improvement in general appearance helps to add to self-esteem. Ultraviolet light must be used with caution and special care must be taken to note a patient's drug regimen because of the photosensitising effect of some drugs (*see* Chapter 6).

A Quiet Treatment Room

A quiet treatment room may be sound-proofed if it is to be used for individual relaxation sessions. The window should be curtained and the decor subdued. The room should have at least one easy chair and be usable as a retreat if a patient needs extra privacy. The room should be warm but with adequate ventilation and the couch in the room wide enough for a patient to relax without fear of falling off and should ideally be of adjustable height. Aids to relaxation might include a tape recorder, soothing music, blank tapes, and possibly a biofeedback machine.

The Office

The physiotherapy office should be large enough for all the staff. It may have to double as a changing room. Apart from the usual office facilities a good range of reference books is essential. The professional library of a psychiatric hospital may carry many of the latest books on mental health care but is unlikely to carry basic texts on the care of fractures, orthopaedic conditions, nerve injuries or many other common medical conditions. If the hospital is in an isolated situation the physiotherapist is advised to maintain a well stocked shelf of basic physical care books. In addition basic psychiatry books are necessary for quick reference.

Catalogues of all kinds of equipment and aids should be stocked in order to give advice when needed.

Files of interesting articles on various psychiatric illnesses and treatments, especially if applicable to physiotherapy, can be gradually compiled for future reference.

The Store

The store should be large enough to accommodate any electrical equipment under lock and key as fire raisers are a hazard in psychiatric hospitals. Useful things to remember to stock which psychiatric wards often do not carry are crepe bandages and sputum pots. Specialist stores may include:

Splint-making equipment
Foam for collars
Plaster scissors
Hand saw
Adjustable spanner
Set of screwdrivers
Bicycle pump
Ferrules
Elasticated tubular bandages
Walking aids.

Many other individual items will of course be stocked as needed.

Toilet Facilities

It may seem rather obvious to state that a patient's toilet in a physiotherapy department should have adequate wheelchair access and that suitable grab rails should be provided, but not so in a psychiatric unit. To illustrate the point a recently upgraded psychogeriatric ward was completed without any provision for grab rails or aids in toilets or bathrooms simply because the staff concerned were looking at the patients from a psychiatric point of view and physical needs were overlooked. It was not until the physiotherapist was shown round the nearly completed unit that anyone realised the omission, everything looked beautiful and homely, but there was not one toilet that could take a wheelchair and partitions between compartments were too weak to take grab rails. The physiotherapist wished she had involved herself at the outset of the project.

Waiting Area

Some form of informal waiting area is desirable even if it is very small. This area can be used to display posters and pamphlets with general health care and keep fit themes. It can be used for informal meetings with relatives and patients, and provide an area for patients needing to take a rest between activities.

The Psychogeriatric Department

The physiotherapy department in a psychogeriatric unit will not need the comprehensive range of gymnastic equipment required for the younger groups of patients; nevertheless the large activity area is still of major importance. Elderly patients need more space to accommodate wheelchairs and easy chairs as well as space for exercise in standing. Groups may vary from a few patients to perhaps a whole ward of say twenty people plus a large number of helpers. A large variety of suitable chairs with arms is necessary together with plenty of walking aids of differing types.

Warmth is especially important for the old, and large high-ceilinged rooms can be cold and draughty. In such rooms an echo can also be confusing for patients; thus the large activity area in a specifically designed psychogeriatric unit needs a lower ceiling than that in a general department and furnishings such as curtains or even washable carpet tiles to dampen the echo.

General equipment will be similar to that already described with the exclusion of the more active gymnastic equipment and the inclusion of as many games as possible which can be played from a chair.

Music for the older patient is chosen with care to include Second and First World War tunes, party songs and dances, Christmas music when appropriate and even children's actions songs. Popular classical works are also appreciated by many especially as ward radios and televisions are often blaring out modern popular music all day.

Wide plinths are necessary in the psychogeriatric unit to allay fears of falling. These should be adjustable in height. Practise stairs may prove useful and as long a stretch of parallel bars as is feasible.

Reality Orientation

The department in a psychogeriatric unit should reinforce the practice of reality orientation which will be in use on the wards and in the day units. The patient is reminded of the basics of day-to-day living with as much stimulation as possible—verbal, visual and tactile. In the physiotherapy department, for example, the patients' toilet and the way out should be clearly labelled in bold lettering. Arrows should point the way and where applicable a picture or sign be displayed.

A long mirror close to the main door can be used to draw a patient's attention to himself and his appearance both on arrival and departure. A clear poster with the date and season can also be displayed.

When talking to confused patients a clear speech and directions must be used, reinforcing the instruction given in as many ways as possible, asking the patient to touch an object, repeat its name and how to use it in an effort to retain the memory for basic essentials. Constant repetition of simple routines helps the failing memory to cope.

Reminiscence Therapy

Reminiscene therapy helps patients who are confused by reminding them of the past they knew. Old people readily remember the past and when the present is all confusion then remembering the past can help to bring a feeling of stability and familiarity. This helps to reduce some of the agitation and insecurity brought on by confusion and a calmer patient can cope better with day-to-day living. All kinds of stimuli are used in reminiscence therapy: old photographs, objects from the past, music and sound and talking about the old days. Pictures on the walls in the physiotherapy department, the music used for group work and above all listening and talking to patients about their past all help to add a feeling of security and to create a pleasurable atmosphere for cooperation in treatment.

The Role of the Physiotherapy Helper

The physiotherapy helper, a very useful person especially in a psychogeriatric unit, is probably under-utilised in many departments because of the lack of general training available to physiotherapy helpers. The helper probably spends most of her time in direct contact with the patient and must be a good communicator.

The physiotherapist responsible for training a helper will currently train the helper for the needs of the department she works in but the helper should also be aware of the role of the whole of the mental health care team of which she is a part. Use can be made, where possible, of in-service training courses for equivalent personnel such as nursing auxiliaries and occupational therapy helpers.[2] The helper working in psychiatry needs to understand not only the basis of the physical treatments and conditions she will encounter but of the psychiatric treatments and conditions too. The teaching of lifting is especially important for helpers who are often required to help with the heaviest patients.

The work of the physiotherapy helper needs careful monitoring by the physiotherapist but it can greatly extend the amount of preventive and recreational work undertaken in a physiotherapy department.

Work which directly involves the helper in the treatment of patients can include:

Helping to lead movement groups while the physiotherapist concentrates on individuals in the group
Organising recreational games groups or music groups
Organising dancing

Routine walking with patients at risk of becoming immobile

Regular checking of patients' hands which are at risk of becoming contracted

Taking patients outside into the grounds

Practising reality orientation

Practising reminiscence therapy

Helping patients dress and undress and preparing them for treatment

Sitting and talking with patients who are unpredictable or need constant monitoring during treatments such as heat treatment or postural drainage

Helping with heavy patients where two or more are needed to lift

Chaperoning during the treatment of patients who may be aggressive. These patients are invariably the confused elderly who may pinch, squeeze, bite or pull hair and may need gentle restraining. If, for example, the physiotherapist is stretching a patient's painful hand in order to maintain enough mobility in the fingers to cut the nails, then the physiotherapy helper may need to hold the patient's other hand to prevent the physiotherapist being struck.

The regular checking of patients' walking aids and wheelchairs for damage or wear. Damage to walking aids is common on units where aggressive patients are housed. The damage is often perpetrated by people other than the user of the aid. Wheelchairs are also vulnerable to abuse.

Other work for the helper which does not directly involve patient contact could include:

Care of apparatus

Setting out apparatus for classwork and treatments

Keeping registers and numbers up to date and helping with general clerical work

Ordering stores, changing linen and other routine department work as needed.

In many departments the helper may have other roles perhaps involving a particular talent, such as the ability to play a musical instrument or sing, which can be utilised in group work. In conclusion, the physiotherapy helper who is well trained and supervised can supplement the overall work of a busy physiotherapy service with great benefit.

The Teaching Role of the Physiotherapist

The increasing importance of the physiotherapist's role in preventive medicine requires all physiotherapists to be teachers. One of the greatest areas of need is in the field of mental health care where the requirements and responses of the body may be overlooked. No patient has ever crossed the portals of a mental hospital bringing his mind with him and leaving his body at home and yet the staff of mental health care teams may pay little attention to body responses.

The physiotherapist who is prepared to spend time teaching will, in the long run, benefit more patients than the physiotherapist who merely treats cases as they present to her.

Self Education Within Psychiatry

Few physiotherapists working in mental health care are as educated in the subject as they would wish to be. The subject is currently one for postgraduate education and the individual physiotherapist must be motivated to attend as many lectures and courses as possible. Most mental health care units run regular lectures for staff which both provide basic revision work and insight into new ideas. The recent formation of a group of physiotherapists with a special interest in psychiatry in the United Kingdom[3] has done much to coordinate the work of isolated physiotherapists and the group now runs regular courses. The Association of Chartered Physiotherapists in Psychiatry regularly organises introductory courses for physiotherapists interested in psychiatric care as well as more advanced courses for those with more experience.

Teaching Qualified Physiotherapists

Physiotherapists working in areas other than that of mental health care will need to know more about mental illness as the mentally ill move into the community. It is possible that community physiotherapists will feel this need most. The teaching must be by those with experience in the subject and the problem can be tackled in the following ways:

> Basic grade physiotherapists should follow a rotation which includes a period in an established physiotherapy department in a mental health care setting.
> Physiotherapists working in mental health care should be prepared to give talks at local group and branch meetings. If necessary the initiative of suggesting a lecture should come from the individual physiotherapist.
> A basic course in psychiatric work should be regularly offered as a postgraduate option in all health districts.

Teaching Physiotherapy Students

Physiotherapy students should have a basic knowledge of the common areas of mental illness and the way in which they affect the body. Detailed knowledge of mental illness is probably best left to postgraduate interests except in the field of psychogeriatrics. The mentally ill elderly are increasing in number and so are their physical problems. Psychogeriatric care should be an essential part of the physiotherapy students training programme.

Teaching Other Professions

Professions trained in and wholly associated with, the care of the mentally ill are largely ignorant of the nature and scope of physical therapy in relation to mental illness. The physical needs of patients are not always recognised or understood. The physiotherapist who is prepared to teach basic physical rehabilitation particularly to nursing staff and demonstrate how its use improves the lifestyle of patients is valued. General lectures can be given to all professional groups but it is the nursing staff who need to know and accept the aims of physical therapy more than any other group, and be motivated to put into practice what is being taught by the physiotherapist for patients' physical problems to improve. Four methods of teaching other professions are suggested.

1 Student psychiatric nurse courses usually include time for lectures from other professions working in the field, and physiotherapy should be one of them. Especially helpful is a lecture in the physiotherapy department prior to a placement studying and nursing psychogeriatric patients. Student nurses can then explore the department and try apparatus. They should be taught:

How to walk with a patient, where to give support and how to use a walking aid
How to teach a patient to turn and sit in safety
How to help a patient to cough and produce phlegm for a sputum specimen
How to position patients with contractures and how to use positioning to prevent contracture
How to move patients through a full range of passive movements to help prevent contractures. This can then be done by a nurse when a patient is relaxing in a bath.

Many nurses may not have seen x-rays of simple fractures which they nurse. The fractured neck of femur is the most common and x-rays showing various prostheses and pins and plates *in situ* always generate interest.

2 Specific physical problems which occur can often be dealt with by a short discussion at a nurses' handover session. Thus if a patient suffers a stroke on a ward where no one has had any recent experience of this type of problem the physiotherapist can teach specific physical management to that ward team at handover time.

3 Trouble shooting sessions with charge nurses are stimulating. Study days for senior nursing staff may be arranged as part of in-service training at a unit. A useful exercise is a trouble shooting session where both senior physiotherapist and senior nurses highlight relevant problems which they are having and discuss how to rectify them.

4 Medical staff and other groups often run courses of lectures and the physiotherapist must be prepared to push for the inclusion of her lectures on the role of physiotherapy in mental health care.

Teaching Patients

Wherever practicable patients need to know about the reactions and the care of their bodies. Patients respond best if they understand the logical basis of treatment and clear explanations should precede treatment. This is not always feasible, as in the case of dementia, but where verbal communication is not possible then touch may be understood. A general improvement in body care and physical fitness helps to reduce the long-term physical problems of the mentally ill.

Teaching Relatives

The relatives of the mentally ill and in particular those caring at home for the mentally ill elderly frequently feel isolated and despairing. A relatives support group may be organised by a member of the mental health care team such as the psychologist or occupational therapist attached to a psychogeriatric unit. The physiotherapist should be known by the relatives who attend the group and should give short talks to the group on subjects such as simple mobility problems, positioning, contracture, and lifting.

The physiotherapist working in the community will be in a position to give on the spot advice and it is to be hoped that those based at a day-centre or with a specific team would be in a position to visit at home if necessary.

Teaching How to Lift

The physiotherapist may find herself under considerable pressure to teach how to lift to staff throughout the hospital. This could be a full time occupation. The amount of lifting the physiotherapist is prepared to teach will depend on the individual situation. It can be very useful to the physiotherapist to be included in the introductory course for nursing helpers and students as this gives the physiotherapist an opportunity to meet newcomers at the start of their training and promote the message of good physical care. Newcomers can also be encouraged to come forward and be involved when they meet the physiotherapist on the wards and in the day centres.

One important point should be made about the teaching of lifting in psychiatric hospitals. The use of the orthodox lift is discouraged by most institutions; the shoulder lift is preferred because it reduces the strain on the back. The shoulder lift is a bad lift to use with some psychiatric patients particularly the aggressive confused elderly. The lifters cannot watch the patient's face and are therefore vulnerable to hair pulling or punching. Staff must be advised to choose the type of lift with care taking into account the mental state of a patient. If in doubt a third person should be asked to help even if the lift would normally only take two.

Treating Staff

There are two schools of thought on treating staff who need a course of physiotherapy. One school says that if staff are treated in the department working time is saved and time off for sickness is reduced, it also improves staff/physiotherapist relationships. The second arises particularly where departments are very short staffed, and is that the physiotherapists are employed to treat the patients. In a large hospital with only one physiotherapist it would be possible to spend more time treating staff than patients. The policy must be decided at a local level.

Research

The benefits of physiotherapy in a mental health care setting are not yet backed by reliable research. There is a need for long-term evaluation of treatments and their effects on patients. In a busy department it is difficult to embark upon a time consuming research project but if physiotherapists do not evaluate their work and prove its worth then in times of economic stringency they may find themselves unemployed. So much is happening in the field of psychiatry that there are ample opportunities to set up pilot studies into the benefits of physical therapy particularly in new community schemes. It is to be hoped that many will take up this challenge and show that what is on offer is of proven benefit.

References

1. The Cinderella Service (1985). *Physiotherapy*, **71(8):** 367.
2. Mead J., Crawford M. and Wells J. Training for helpers—a multidisciplinary approach. *Physiotherapy*, **71(8):** 355.
3. Mead P. (1985) Psychiatry. In: *Chartered Physiotherapists' Source Book*, p. 192. Parke Sutton Publishing in association with The Chartered Society of Physiotherapy, 14 Bedford Row, London WC1.

Appendix I

Movement Therapy Sources

The use of various movement therapies has been advocated in this book with the aims of promoting general physical and mental well being, self esteem, self awareness, awareness of others, communication with others, self expression and relaxation. A wide variety of movement resources are available and those used will vary according to the interests of the patients, the physiotherapists and the facilities available. The chronically sick will become bored if the same routines are produced week after week, thus it is important for the physiotherapist to familiarise herself with as many alternatives as possible and to be aware of what others are offering. Above all movement sessions should be fun, if the work is not enjoyed by the participants then the aims of the work will not be achieved.

General Reading

Bassey E. J., Fentem P. H. (1981). *Exercise—The Facts*. Oxford: Oxford University Press.

Berne E. (1964). *Games People Play*. Harmondsworth: Penguin Books.

Department of Education and Science, Safety Series No 4 (1978). *Safety in Physical Education*. London: HMSO.

Latto K. (1981). *Give Us the Chance. Sport and Recreation with Mentally Handicapped People*. The Disabled Living Foundation, 346 Kensington High Street, London W14 8NS.

Straub W. F. (1980). *Sport Psychology*. Chester: Mouvement Publications.

Organisations Providing General Information on Aspects of Movement, Fitness and Health

Central Council for Physical Recreation
Francis House, Francis Street, London WC1A 1AH.

Health Education Council
78 New Oxford Street,
London WC1A 1AH.

The Disabled Living Foundation
346 Kensington High Street,
London N14 8NS.

The Sports Council
70 Brompton Road, London SW3 1EX.

Keep Fit and Training Techniques

'Keep fit' is big business in the western world today. Fitness centres and classes are appearing in every town, some are run by well qualified experts, others are organised by people with minimal knowledge and training in the field of physical fitness. It is often hard for the general public to discern which is which, but very important that vulnerable people such as the mentally ill are in the capable hands of those who are properly trained, such as teachers of physical education, physiotherapists and remedial gymnasts.

Keep fit is often associated with slimming programmes and such classes are given names like 'slimobility' or 'tone and trim'. Well organised groups run by properly trained instructors have a great deal to offer the overweight person, but once again extremist diets and gimmicks have to be avoided. Whatever fancy name is given to these groups and whether they use music, dance, groupwork or other techniques they are all basically 'keep fit' which implies the maintenance of a good general level of physical fitness.

Training, on the other hand, implies something more than just keeping fit. It implies pushing the body on to achieve additional physical strength and endurance beyond that normally needed to suit a person's particular lifestyle. Training is often undertaken in order to perform at a better level in a particular sport and the muscle work done is very specific. Sometimes musculature is developed to extremes for the sake of appearances by body builders, this is known popularly as 'pumping'. Once again many private gymnasia exist, some providing expert trained instructors and others minimal assistance. The multigym which can be used by several people at once in a relatively small area is very popular and is used in many units which care for the mentally ill.

Further Reading

Cook S., Toms A. (1973). *Royal Marine Commando 7 Exercises*. London: Sphere Books Ltd.

Fowler E. (1983). *Keep Fit*. Essex, Laughton: Judy Piatkus (Publishers).

Morgan R. E., Adamson G. T. (1961). *Circuit Training*. London: Bell and Hyman.

Ross K. (1973). *The New Manual of Yoga*. Berkshire, Slough: W. Foulsham & Co. Ltd.

Sorensen J., Bruns W. (1979). *Aerobic Dancing*. Australia, Sydney: Angus Robertson Publishers.

Tancred W., Tancred G. (1984). *Weight Training for Sport*. Kent, Sevenoaks: Hodder and Stoughton Educational Books.

Organisations

British Amateur Weight Lifting Association
3 Iffley Turn,
Oxford

British Wheel of Yoga
445 High Road,
Ilford, Essex

Keep Fit Association
70 Brompton Road,
London SW3 1HE

Local Community Adult Education Centres and
Colleges of Further Education

Medau Society of Great Britain
8b Robson House, East Street,
Epsom, Surrey KT17 1HH

Womans League of Health and Beauty
30 Artillary Lane,
London E1 72T

Creative Movement

Creative movement is one of the most exciting areas in which to work with the mentally ill with its potential for self expression and body awareness. Creative movement is based largely on the teachings of Rudolf Laban and from these creative movement activities have developed those involving dance, music, mime and drama. With regard to drama, its use in movement activities must not be confused with *Psychodrama*. Psychodrama is a psychotherapeutic technique used in specialised group therapy sessions in which the subject is encouraged to act out a significant happening in his past with other members of the group taking relevant roles in the drama. This type of drama can only be supervised by fully trained therapists in psychodrama as it often leads to the release of deep emotional reactions. *Drama Therapy* can be used however to help a person act out a particular problem he has in communicating with others such as entering a crowded room or asking the way when lost.

Further Reading

Anderson M. E. (1970). *Inventive Movement*. Edinburgh: Chambers.
Barker C. (1977). *Theatre Games*. London: Methuen.
Bartal L., Ne'eman N. (1975). *Movement Awareness and Creativity*. London: Souvenir Press.

Exiner J., Lloyd P. (1974). *Teaching Creative Movement*. Lewes, Sussex: New Educational Press Ltd.
Hamblin K. (1978). *Mime*. California, San Francisco: Headlands Press Inc.
Schulberg C. H. (1981). *The Music Therapy Source Book*. New York: Human Sciences Press Inc.
Smedley R., Tether J. (1972). *Let's Dance—Country Style*. London: Paul Elek Books Ltd.
Preston-Dunlop. (1980). *A Handbook for Dance in Education*. Plymouth: Macdonald and Evans.

Organisations

British Society for Music Therapy
48 Lanchester Road,
London N6 4TA

Imperial Society of Teachers of Dancing
Euston Hall, Birkenhead Street,
London WC1H 8BE

Laban Art of Movement Guild
Mullions, Eastcombe, Stroud,
Gloucester GL6 7EA

SESAME (Movement and Drama)
Christchurch, 27 Blackfriars Road,
London SE1 8NI

Indoor and Outdoor Sports, Games and Pastimes

Sports and games are pursued as much for social reasons as for physical gain. Sport therefore is a means of communicating and cooperating with others in a recreational way and has much to offer the mentally ill. A sporting activity pursued in a hospital or day centre can be taken up in the community and provide companionship and purposeful recreation. The pursuit of a sport coincidentally helps to keep the body fit and healthy. The relaxation of mind and body provided by a sport is another important aspect, especially for those who have stressful but sedentary jobs. The use of a tension control technique may provide the answer to problems of stress while at work but a recreational physical pursuit may be a better method of relaxation at home.

When introducing sporting activities to people who not only have mental problems but who may not have played a team game since leaving school, simplicity and enjoyment are the key to retaining a continued interest in playing a sport. The excellent books which are produced for teaching school children are full of simple indoor and outdoor activities which are fun, develop movement skills and would be enjoyed as much by adults as they are by children. Mini versions of major sports are also popular. They are designed to be played in small areas, have simplified rules and need fewer numbers of people than the full game.

It is not necessary for a sporting activity to be competitive and some people dislike this element of sport, for them the more individual pursuits may be more suitable. Activities such as jogging, riding, swimming and rambling can all provide exercise and companionship.

Further Reading

Elkington H. (1978). *Swimming, A Handbook for Teachers*. Cambridge: Cambridge University Press.

Croucher N. (1981). *Outdoor Pursuits for Disabled People*. Cambridge: Woodhead-Faulkner Ltd.

Know the Game Series. A series of titles covering major sports and games. Wakefield: E. P. Publishing Ltd.

Parratt A. L. (1983). *Indoor Games and Activities*. London: Hodder and Stoughton.

Reid-Campion M. (1985). *Hydrotherapy in Paediatrics*. London: William Heinemann Medical Books.

Royal Life Saving Society (1978). *Life Saving*. London: Royal Life Saving Society.

Sleap M. (1984). *Mini Sport*. London: Heinemann Educational Books.

Wise W. M. (1983). *Games and Sports*. London: Heinemann Educational Books.

Organisations

Amateur Swimming Association
Harold Fern House, Derby Square,
Loughborough, Leicester LE11 0AC

British Sports Association for the Disabled
Sir Ludwig Guttman Sports Centre, Harvey Road,
Aylesbury, Bucks

National Jogging Association
35 Bruton Street,
London W1X 7DD

Riding for the Disabled
Avenue R, National Agricultural Centre,
Stoneleigh, Kenilworth,
Warwicks CV8 2LY.

Movement for the Elderly

The maintenance of fitness through movement is increasingly important as people live longer lives. The mentally ill elderly are at great risk of suffering additional hardships through immobility. Once the physiotherapist has made appropriate allowances for individual infirmity and stamina then keep fit and creative movement work are very beneficial. Whilst the most active sports and games are no longer appropriate for the majority, some games such as table tennis, bowls and circle ball games are much enjoyed.

Music selected for older people should reflect their tastes and interests, modern popular music is not usually appreciated but neither is an unending supply of 'knees up' type party dances. Where possible people should be encouraged to select their own choice of music. Many older people are skilled ballroom dancers and this art can be enjoyed well on into extreme old age. Now it is regrettable that as younger generations age they will not be able to draw on this skill for recreation.

Adult education centres frequently offer specialised fitness classes for the elderly. Sometimes these classes are associated with some form of social or lunch club. Such clubs could provide much needed companionship for an elderly person attempting to recover from a mental illness.

Further Reading

Caplow Linder E., Harpaz L., Samberg S. (1979). *Therapeutic Dance/Movement*. Expressive activities for older adults. London: Human Science Press.

Organisations

EXTEND (Exercise Training for the Elderly and Disabled)
Conway House, 5 Conway Road,
Sheringham, Norfolk NR2 8DD

Local Authority and Community Adult Education Centres

Massage and Other Body Orientated Therapies

The use of massage as a healing technique can be traced back in time to the origins of health care techniques in many cultures. The physiotherapist should draw on her skills as a masseuse in the treatment of the mentally ill particularly those patients suffering from stress or tension. The use of touch as a means of communication is brought to the fore through massage and massage techniques are an important component of some body orientated psychotherapeutic techniques.

There are a number of so called 'new therapies' used both within traditional psychiatric practice and independently of it. Many of these practices use the body or massage as a vehicle for self expression and intercommunication. The physiotherapist is unlikely to be involved in practising these therapies unless specifically trained to do so, however she would be wise to read about such therapies and be aware of the other areas of treatment in which patients may be involving themselves. Some techniques may seem bizarre, others may have relevance for the physiotherapist, all should be viewed with an open inquiring mind.

Fashions in health care change, and it is only a few years since the idea of a physiotherapist practising acupuncture would have been regarded as unacceptable, now recognised training courses are available. New techniques and alternative therapies should neither be accepted nor condemned out of ignorance or prejudice.

Further Reading

Drury N. (1984). *The Bodywork Book*. Prism Alpha Ltd, Church House, Half Moon Street, Sherborne, Dorset DT9 3LN

Lewith G. (ed). (1985). *Alternative Therapies*. London: William Heinemann Medical Books.

Liss J. (1974). *Free to Feel*. London: Wildwood House Ltd, 1 Wardour Street, London.

Appendix II

Useful Addresses

Age Concern
Bernard Sunley House, 60 Pitcairn Road,
Mitcham, Surrey CR4 3LL

Alzheimer's Disease Society
Bank Buildings, Fulham Broadway,
London SE6 1EP

Association to Combat Huntingtons Choroea (COMBAT)
Theydon Road, Epping,
Essex CM16 4DX

British Epilepsy Association
Crowthorne House, New Wokingham Road,
Wokingham, Berks

Disabled Living Foundation
346 Kensington High Street,
London W14 8NS

Help the Aged
32 Dover Street,
London W1A 2AP

Mental Health Foundation
8 Wimpole Street, London W1M 8HY

MIND (National Association for Mental Health)
22 Harley Street, London

Multiple Sclerosis Society of Great Britain and Northern Ireland
4 Tachbrook Street,
London SW1V 1SJ

National Council for Carers and their Elderly Dependants
29 Chilworth Mews,
London W2 3RG

National Schizophrenia Fellowship
78–79 Victoria Road,
Surbiton, Surrey

Parkinson's Disease Society of the UK Ltd.
81 Queens Road,
London SW19 8NR

SESAME
27 Blackfriar's Road, London SE1 8NY

The Schizophrenia Association of Great Britain
Llanfair Hall, Caernarfon,
Gwynedd LL55 1TT

Index

acetylcholine levels, 110
aches, treatment of, 54, 55
activity equipment, in physiotherapy department, 160–1
acute
  mental disorders, common, 17–39
  mental illness unit, 12–17
  organic psychoses, 7, 73
  schizophrenia, 36, 55
addiction, 130–9
  to alcohol, 130, 131–8
  to drugs, 130, 138–9
  to glue and solvents, 139
    case history, 140
  to nicotine, 130
admission to psychiatric unit
  compulsory, 2
  sections of Mental Health Acts governing, 3, 129, 141
addresses of organisations, 183, 184
adolescent units, 154, 159
affective disorders, classified, 6–8
agoraphopia, 29
  initiation of, 109–10
aids to mobility, 50, 88, 105, 147, 161, 167
  case history, 51, 52
alcohol abuse, 7, 129–38
alcohol addiction
  chronic, 131
  treatment of, 132–8
alcohol addiction unit, 134, 135
alcoholic dementia, 134, 137
  case history, 137–8
Alexander Technique, the, 118
Alzheimer-type disease (senile dementia), 7, 67–71
  case history, 69–70
amputation, 65
anorexia nervosa, 7, 33–4
anoxia, effects of, 22, 63, 73
antianxiety drugs, 94, 100
  dependency on, 101
  major groups of, 100–1
anticholinergic drugs, 96, 103
anticonvulsant drugs, 94, 106
antidepressant drugs, 94
  side-effects of, 95–100
antiparkinsonian drugs, 94, 102
  case history, 105-6
  side-effects of, 103, 104
antipsychotic drus, 94, 101
  administration of, 103
  generic groups of, 101
  side-effects of, 101–3, 104
anxiety neuroses, 5, 108–9
anxiety states, 7, 25, 27
  case history, 27–8
  drugs prescribed for, 95, 101
  in elderly, 77
  physical assessment of, 26

physical symptoms of, 25, 112–13
anxiolytics, 100
appeal, patients' rights of, 2
arthritic knees, 83
arthritis, rheumatoid, 8, 76
assessment, physical, 82
assessment ward, psycho-geriatric, 81–5
accidents on, 82
Association of Chartered Physiotherapists in Psychiatry, 168
asthma, 8, 48, 113
asylum, 1, 5
atmosphere, of physiotherapy department, 158
autonomic nervous system, 25, 110, 111
brain centres controlling, 110

ballroom dancing, as therapy, 180, 181
barbiturates, 100, 139
bath, wax, 161
bedsores, 88
behaviour therapy, 9
for phobias, 115
behavioural units, 155
bereavement, 76
beta-blocking agent, 101
biofeedback machines, 125
biological depression, 19
blurred vision, as anxiety symptom, 112
as side-effect of drugs, 97
Bobath techniques, 60
body language, 113
signs of tension, 113, 114
brain confusion, acute, 7
brain damage, 7
case history, 63
following anoxia, 22, 63
from head injury, 62–4
in epilepsy, 57
permanent, 7
brain trauma, 7
breathing
disturbed, as anxiety symptom, 124
exercises, 20
British National Formulary, 94, 97
bulimia, 7
butyrophenones, 101

cardiovascular disorders, 8
case histories given on
alcoholic dementia, 137
alcoholic dependency, 136–7
agoraphobia, 109
anxiety states, 27–8, 108–9
brain damage, 63
chronic schizophrenia, 56, 57
concealed disability, 76
debility, in depression, 20–1, 76–7, 98–9
drug side-effects, 98–9, 105–6
epilepsy, 55, 58
glue sniffing, 40
head injury, 63–4
Huntington's Chorea, 59, 60, 61
hyperventilation, 27–8, 78
hysteria, 31–2
manic depressive psychosis, 24–5, 55
mobility aids, 51, 52
pain, 55, 83
physical injury, in chronic mental illness, 53, 55, 56–7
schizophrenia, 38–9, 56–7

self-esteem, 15–16, 48–9
self-inflicted injury, 23
senile dementia, 69–73
severe debility, 20–2
steroid-induced psychosis, 17
tardive dyskinesia, 105
touch communication, 127
cerebral anoxia, 7
chairs
  for long-stay wards, 89
  wheel, 50, 51, 88
chaperoning, of aggressive patient, 167
chest disease, 54, 77, 135
chest infection, 20
  in elderly, 77, 83, 84
children's unit, 156
chronic mental illness, 41–65
  and community care, 41
  in the elderly, 42, 43
  in the young, 42, 48, 61, 86
  physical problems of, 52–65
  treatment of, 46–65
chronic organic psychoses, 7
chronic schizophrenia, 55–7
chronically mentally ill
  provision for, 9
  young, 86
clinical psychologist, 9
colitis, 8
communication
  case history, 127
  importance of, 126, 127
  through speech, 23, 24
  through touch, 23
  via movement therapy, 174
  with mental health care team, 12, 27, 37, 85, 169
community care
  physiotherapy services, 80, 91–3
  policy for mentally ill elderly, 92
  therapeutic, 46
  treatment, 3, 4
  work, 44–6
compulsive states, obsessive, 7
compulsory admission, to institutions, 2, 129, 141
confusional states, toxic, 73
contracted hands, 89, 167
contractures, 73, 88
  contrast, relaxation technique (Jacobsen technique), 116
conversion hysteria, 30–2
coronary heart disease, 8
creative movement, 177
  additional information sources on, 178
crime, and mental illness, 142–3
cuddling, as therapy, 127

dance, as therapy, 166, 177, 178
day care, 91–3
day centres, 44–6, 80, 90–2, 171
debility
  case histories, 20–2, 76–7
  in depressed elderly, 76
  severe, 20
delirium, 7, 73
delusion, and criminal acts, 142
dementia
  alcoholic, 134–8
  pseudo depressive, 75
  senile, 67–73
dependence
  on alcohol, chronic, 131
  on drugs, (prescribed), 99, 101
depression, 7, 18, 67, 74–84
  biological, 19

case history, 23, 24
in elderly, 74–84
manic, 24, 75, 95
neurotic, 7, 95–6
physical problems of, 19
psychotic, 19, 76
symptom clusters of, 18, 19
depressive psychosis, manic, 24, 75, 85
case history, 24–5
physical assessment of, 24
detention, of psychiatric patient
compulsory, 2
section orders for, 3, 141–2, 145
diabetes mellitus, 8
diet, and MAOI drugs, 98
diplegia, spastic, 72
disability, concealed, 76
dizziness, as anxiety symptom, 112
drama therapy, 177, 178
drinking problem unit, 134, 135
drug
abuse, 7
addiction, 130, 138–9
addiction treatment centres, 139
interactions, 94, 100, 106, 107
therapy
alternative to, 19, 94, 95
extreme reaction to, 107
for elderly depressed, 75
sensitivity of elderly to, 107
steroid, 17
drug-induced problems, 55, 102
drugs, of addiction
classification of, 139
prescription of, 139
drugs, psychiatric
and diet, 98
and weight gain, 98, 99
dependency on, 99, 101
habit-forming, 100
interactions between, 94, 100, 106, 107
main groups of, 94, 100, 101, 106
prescribed for the elderly, 107
psychotropic, 94–107
side-effects of, 19, 42, 47, 84, 94–107

eating disorders, 7
eczema, 8
elderly, the
comprehensive phsyiotherapy service for, 79
community care for, 91, 92
depressed, 74–9
mentally ill, 66–93
on antidepressant drugs, 97
electroconvulsive therapy (ECT), 10, 75, 77, 84
electroplexy, 10
emotional disturbance, and physical illness, 8
epilepsy, 7, 41, 57, 100, 106, 155
Association, 183
case history, 58
equipment, for physiotherapy department, 160–2
extrapyramidal symptoms, 101–2, 104–6
as lesions, 104
case history, 105–6
drug-induced, 104

family therapy, 10

'fight or flight' reaction, 108, 110
files, on psychiatric illnesses, 162
fitness
　classes, for the elderly, 181
　programmes, 150
forensic
　psychiatry, 140–3
　unit, regional, 144
Freud S., 9
functional psychoses, 6
furniture, on long-stay wards, 89, 90

gastritis, in alcohol dependents, 134
gastrointestinal disorders, 8
glue sniffing, 139, 140
'grand mal' seizure, 58
group
　homes, 9, 10
　therapy, 44
　work, 54
gymnasium facilities, 48
gymnast, remedial, 47

habit-forming drugs, 100
hay fever, 8
head injury, 62
headache, as anxiety symptom, 112
heart disease
　and stress control, 115
　effect of tricyclic antidepressants on, 97
heat
　pack, flexible, 161
　lamps, 161
hemiplegia, 76
holiday relief ward, 90
holistic medicine, 8

hospital
　order, under Mental Health Act, 141
　psychiatric, 42, 43
　special, 144, 151
Huntington's Chorea, 7, 41, 58–62, 73
hypertension, 8
hyperthyroidism, 8
hyperventilation, 15, 25, 77, 96, 113
　case history, 27–8, 78
　syndrome, 124
　treatment of, 124
hypnosis, 118
hypoxia, 124
hysteria, 7, 30
　conversion, 30–2
　mass, 30

imagery, relaxation therapy, 123
impotence, as anxiety symptom, 107
inferential therapy unit, 161
injury, self-inflicted, 22
　head, 62–4
insomnia, severe, 100
interaction of psychotic drugs, 107

Jacobsen E., 116, 117
job satisfaction, 93
Jones Maxwell, 46

keep fit
　classes, 175
　routine, 15

Laban Rudolf, 177
Laura Mitchell Method (of relaxation), 117

liaison psychiatry, 11
lifting of patients, 166
　teaching to others, 172
limbic system, 110
lithium carbonate, side-effects, 100
liver disease, 134
long-stay patients, 43, 89
long-term care ward, for elderly, 85
　physiotherapy applications in, 86–90
Lunacy Act 1890, 1

Mad House Act, 1
major tranquillisers, 101–3
mania, 19, 95
manic depressive illness, 24–5, 55, 100–2
　case histories, 24, 55
MAOI drugs, 19, 95, 96, 98, 99
marital therapy, 10
mass hysteria, 30
massage
　as tension reducer, 126, 181
　therapy, 181, 182
meditation, 118
mental crisis, acute, 81
Mental Health Act 1959, 1, 4
　amendments, 2
Mental Health Act 1983, 2, 129
　aims, 2
　regulations governing, 2, 3, 129
　Section 37, 3, 141
　Section 41, 3, 141, 142, 145
Mental Health Act Commission, 3
mental health care, in UK
　currently, 2–5
　historically, 1–2

mental health tribunal, 2
mental illness, 2
　acute, 12, 17–39
　chronic, 41–65
　classified, 6–8
　common terms defined, 8–10
　in the elderly, 20, 66, 93, 180
　　community care for, 91, 92
　　drugs prescribed for, 94–107
　　physiotherapy service for, 79
mental handicap *see* mental impairment
mental impairment, 2, 8, 64
　and criminal acts, 143
　severe, 2
Mental Treatment Act 1930, 1
Misuse of Drugs Act 1971, 139
Misuse of Drugs Regulations 1973, 139
Mitchell, Laura (relaxation method), 117
mobility
　aids, 50, 51, 88, 105, 147
　maintenance of, 86, 87, 167
　monitoring, 86, 88
　movement sessions for, 13, 14, 87, 88, 89, 122, 174, 177
monoamine oxidase inhibitors (MAOI drugs), 19, 95
　and diet, 98, 99
　dependency on, 99
　time factors of, 96
　usage, 95
Monthly Index of Medical Specialties (MIMS), 94
movement therapy, 115, 174
　creative, 177
　for the elderly, 87, 164, 180, 181

Index 191

further information sources on, 174, 177
group sessions, 13, 14, 87, 88, 166, 174
relaxation as, 122–3, 174
multi-infarct dementia, 67, 70–1
case history, 71–3
multigym, 149, 150, 161, 176
multiple sclerosis, 22, 74
Society, 183
music therapy, 166, 177, 178
myopathy, 133

National Association for Mental Health (MIND), 3, 183
nerve and tendon damage (self-inflicted), 22
neuroleptic drugs, 47, 52, 55
neurological conditions, 65
progressive, 60, 73–4
neuropsychiatric units, 155
neuroses
chronic, 41
classified, 6, 7
neurosyphilis, 65, 73
neurotic depression, 7, 95, 96
noradrenaline levels, 110, 112
nurse, psychiatric, 41

obsessional disorders, 7, 9
occupational therapist, 41, 91
Odent, Michel (relaxation techniques), 126
oedema, 97
opiates, 139
opium addicts, 129
organic psychoses, 7

pain, treatment of
as anxiety symptom, 112, 113
in chronically mentally ill, 54, 55
in elderly depressed, 83
Papworth Hospital, Cambridge, 124
and hyperventilation syndrome, 125
paranoid states, in elderly, 79
paraplegia, 22, 65, 98
parasympathetic nervous system, 111–12
Parkinson's Disease, 73
Society for, 84
parkinsonism, 55
case history, 105–6
drug-induced, 102
treatment of, 105
patient information, 171
personality disorders, 41
in elderly, 79
'petit mal' attack, in epilepsy, 57
phenothiazine, 101
phobia (s), 7, 9, 28–30
drugs prescribed for, 95
hospital, 15
initiation of, 109–18
in the elderly, 77
photosensitivity, and psychotic drugs, 103, 148
physical
activity group, 44, 45
assessment, 17
disability, 4, 5
concealed, 75
handicap, 22
independence, 47
problems of ageing, 66
problems, of chronically mentally ill, 52–65
recreation, in secure units, 149–52

therapy, 173
training, 176
physiotherapist, as teacher, 168–72
physiotherapy applications
and mental health, 4, 5
in acute mental illness, 12, 17–39
in chronic mental illness, 46–65
in the community, 80, 91–3, 171
with elderly mentally ill, 66–93
with long-stay patients, 43, 85–90
within specialist units, 128–56
physiotherapy department (in mental health setting)
facilities required in, 162–8
in secure situation, 147, 148, 149
in special hospitals, 151, 152–3
office requirements in, 162
treatment equipment, minimal, 159–64
physiotherapy helper
training of, 166
work of, 166–8
polyneuropathy, 133
Poor Law Act, 1
postural
exercises, 19
hypotension, 96
training, 123
posture, poor, as anxiety symptom, 123
premenstrual tension, 8
pressure sores, 73
propranolol, 100, 101

pseudo dementia, depressive, 75
psychiatric
drugs, side-effects of, 94–107
history, of patient, 18
hospital, 42, 43
nurse, 41
psychiatrist, defined, 8, 9
psychiatry, forensic, 140–3
psychiatry in physiotherapy schools, 5
psychoanalysis, 177
psychodrama, 177
psychogeriatric
assessment ward, 76, 81–5
care, patterns of, 80
day care centre, 80, 91–2
long-stay ward, 85–90
team, 79, 80, 84
unit, 67, 80, 81, 85, 158, 164–8
psychogeriatrician, 66, 72
psychology, defined, 9
psychopath, 147
psychopathy, 142–3
psychoses
acute, organic, 73
classified, 6–7
drug treatment of, 94
major, 41
psychosis, 95, 102
psychosomatic disorders, 2, 8
psychosurgery, 11
psychotherapy, 9, 10, 19, 143
long-term unit, 41
psychotic depression, 19, 76
psychotic drugs, side-effects of, 94–107
psychotrophic drugs, 94–107

reality orientation, 68, 165, 167
recreational activities

in acute unit, 14, 15
in psychogeriatric ward,
  86–8
in special hospitals, 151
reference information,
  essential, 162
regional secure unit, 144–52
relatives' support group, 171
relaxation
  aids, 122–7
  equipment, 160
  group, 121
  in everyday situation, 127,
    128
  methods, 116–19, 125, 126
  teaching, 119, 122–9
  understanding of, 120
  via movement therapy, 174
relaxation therapy
  and anxiety states, 27
  in acute unit, 16
  in day centres, 44
  with chronically mentally ill,
    50, 60
remedial equipment, 160
reminiscence therapy, 165, 167
research into physiotherapy in
  mental health, 5, 173
rheumatoid arthritis, 8, 76
'Rising Tide, The', 66
rollator-type walking aid, 105

schizophrenia, 6, 34, 41, 42, 55,
    147
  acute, 36, 55
  and crime, 142
  chronic, 39, 47, 55, 85
  organisations for, 184
  rehabilitation units for, 41
  treatment for, 35–9, 47, 101,
    102
    case histories, 38–9, 56–7

secure units, 144–50
  physiotherapy in, 149–54,
    159
  violence management in,
    146–7
self-awareness, of patient, 174
self-esteem, of patient, 14, 48,
    174
  case history, 15–16, 48, 49
self expression, in movement
  therapy, 174
self-inflicted injury, 22
  case history, 23, 24
senile dementia, 5, 67–73, 85
severe mental impairment, 2
sexual
  disorders, 7, 101
  offenders, 143
shock therapy, 10
side-effects of psychiatric
  drugs, 94–107
simple phobias, 29
smoking
  among alcohol dependents,
    134
  among chronically mentally
    ill, 54
social
  phobias, 29
  therapy, 41, 42, 43
solvent abuse, 139, 140
specialist units, working in,
    129–56
speech communication, 23, 24
sporting activities, 178, 179
sports equipment, in
    physiotherapy
    department, 160
staff sensitivity groups, 159
steroid drug therapy, 17
steroid-induced psychosis, 17
stress

control techniques, 115–28
illnesses, initiation of, 108–9
physical signs of, 112–14
physiological response to, 110
stress-related disorders, 114–28
student psychiatric nurse, 170
suicidal patient, 5, 22, 23, 74
  elderly, 74
sun beds, 161–2
sunlight
  and photosensitive patient, 103, 148
  importance of, 150
surgical appliances, 51
swimming, as physical outlet, 126
sympathetic nervous system, 110, 111

tabes dorsalis, 65
tapes, for relaxation therapy, 125
tardive dyskinesia, 55
  and antipsychotic drugs, 102, 104
  case history, 105–6
  irreversible, 105
teaching role, of physiotherapist, 168–72
tension, physical signs of, 113–14
terminal care, 90
therapeutic community, the, 46
therapist
  art, 41
  music, 41, 104
  occupational, 41, 47, 84
therapy
  alternative, 182
  behaviour, 9, 155
  drama, 177

drug, 94, 139
electroconvulsive (ECT), 10, 11
group, 9, 10
movement, 13, 14, 87, 122, 174, 177
music, 164, 166, 177, 178
occupational, 41, 47
psycho, 9, 10, 19, 41, 143
reminiscence, 165–6
shock, 10
touch, 23, 126, 181–2
thioxanthenes, 101
toilet facilities, in physiotherapy department, 163
touch communication, 23, 181
  case history, 127
  importance in mental illness, 126
touch withdrawal, 127
toxic confusional states, 73
training
  of physiotherapist, 168, 169
  physical, 176
tranquillisers, 94
  major, 101
treatment area, in physiotherapy department, 161–2
treatment evaluation, 173
tricyclic antidepressant drugs, 95
  and the elderly, 97
  side-effects of, 95–7

ulcers, 8
ultra sound machine, 161
uniform, wearing of, 158
units
  for acute mental illness, 12–39

for chronically mentally ill, 41–3
specialist, 128–56
psychogeriatric, 66–93
useful addresses, listed, 183–4

Vagrancy Act, 1
Valium, 100
violence, in secure unit situation, 146–7
vision blurred,
  as anxiety symptom, 112
  in elderly, 97
voluntary associations, 3

walking aids, 50, 51, 88, 105
  in physiotherapy department, 161, 167
  in secure unit situation, 147

ward team, 12, 13, 15, 18, 22, 47, 74, 99, 104
ward type
  heavy dependency, 43
  hostel, 43
  long-stay, 42, 85–90
warmth, for the elderly, 164
water, as relaxation medium, 125, 126
wax bath, 161
Wernicke-Korsakoff Syndrome, 133
wheelchair access, 163
wheelchairs, 50, 51, 88
  checking of, 167
workshop, sheltered, 43

yoga, 117–18
young chronically sick, provision for, 86